Inside Information

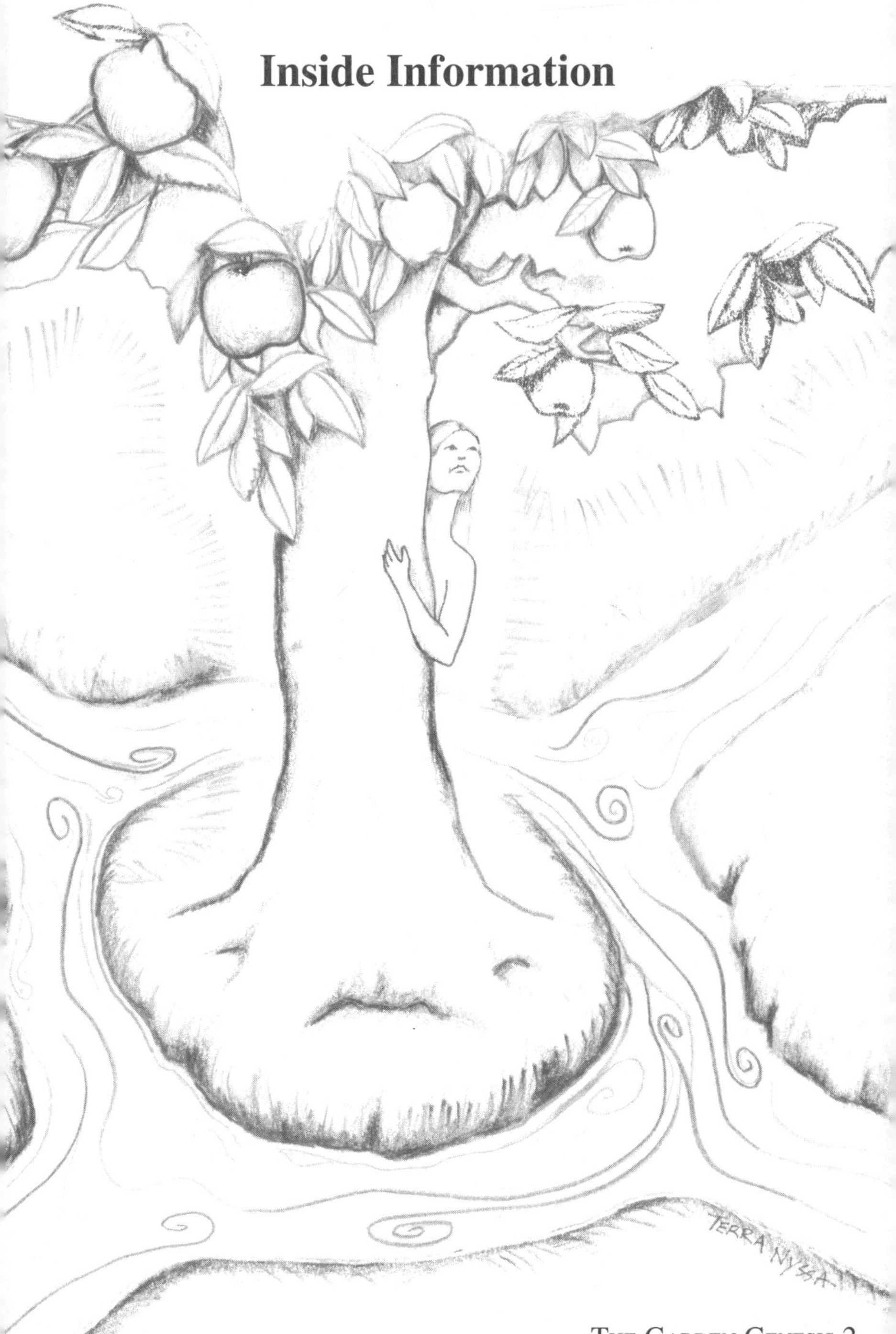

THE GARDEN GENESIS 2

Inside Information:
Life Experiences and the Source of Personal Transformations

Byron Turner

Bay Publishing
BERKELEY, CALIFORNIA

Those interested are invited to write to the author:

Byron Turner
1040 Oak Knoll
Lafayette, Ca 94549 baypub@pacbell.net

Library of Congress Catalogue Card Number: 98-94928

Bay Publishing
Inside Information: Life Experiences and the Source of Personal Transformations
Bibliography
Index

1. Brainsciences. 2. Neurophysiological wholeness. 3. Psychobiological transformations. 4. Religious source hypothesis. 5. God in our brain. 6. Life experiences.

ISBN 0-9669931-0-1

Editor: Paul Weisser, Ph.D.
Frontispiece: Terra Nyssa

Contents

List of Figures, *vii*

Acknowledgments, *ix*

Epigraphs, *xi*

Introduction, *1*

Chapter 1: The Neurostatic Experience, *5*

Chapter 2: Neurostasis—Inside Information, *29*

Chapter 3: Neurostatic Representations, *71*

Chapter 4: Our Brains' Answer, *107*

Chapter 5: Summary and Hypothesis, *115*

Bibliography, *123*

Index, *127*

This book is dedicated to all those who have experienced God, themselves, and their own brain —and more so to those who have not.

List of Figures

Figure 1: Hindu Symbol, *22*

Figure 2: Partial Front View of the Human Brain, *36*

Figure 3: "The Secret Where Four Streets Meet" (1953), painting by the author, *62*

Figure 4: "An Unsuccessful Attempt" (1973), painting by the author, *63*

Figure 5: Untitled Mandala (1920), painting by Carl Jung, *78*

Figure 6: Mandala: "Eternal Window" (1927), painting by Carl Jung, *79*

Figure 7: "Mandala Universe" (1991), by Darryl Reanney, *81*

Figure 8: "Impression of the Artist as Incorporeal Witness to the Center of the Universe" (1979), by Robert Arneson, *84*

Figure 9: Silk and Wool Persian Prayer Rug, *85*

Figure 10: Mandala from West Bhutan, *87*

Figure 11: The Sri Yantra, a Hindu Mandala from India, *88*

Figure 12: Hindu Mandala Bindu, *89*

Figure 13: Bighorn Medicine Wheel, photo by Mark Junge, *91*

Figure 14: A Monstrance of the Roman Catholic Church, *93*

Figure 15: Labyrinth at the California Pacific Medical Center, *94*

Figure 16: Nazi Swastikas on Parade, *96*

Figure 17: St. Peter's Tomb in the Vatican, *98*

Figure 18: Stonehenge, *99*

Figure 19: Boroabuour Stupa in Java, *101*

Figure 20: Earth as Seen from Space (NASA), *102*

Acknowledgments

I wish to thank Beverly Giammara, at the University of Kentucky, for her critical review and suggestions, and Bonny Stevenson for her research. I am grateful to Gail Rauscher, Terra Valentin, and Tran Turner for their early reviews and comments. I was encouraged by Beula Metheney, Arla Green, and Clara Anderson. I especially want to thank my wife Joyce, who suffered through my preoccupation with understanding and helpfulness.

The final manuscript was immensely improved by my editor, Paul Weisser, for which I am very grateful. That some parts of the book are still not easy to read is my fault, not his. In regard to subject matter, I would like to acknowledge the responses received from J. Allan Hobson of Harvard Medical School, Paul D. MacLean of the Department of Health and Human Services, and Walter J. Freeman of the University of California, Berkeley.

Along with many individuals who are woven into my life, I wish to acknowledge Donald Shipley, Raymond Omo, and Robert Sledge. I also want to thank Galen Pumphrey, who initially thought I might have gone crazy when the experience occurred, and the poet Richard Mitchell, who knew what had happened.

With the growing abundance from the Tree of Knowledge or tree of awareness, I would like to include my recognition of Carl Jung, who brought human consciousness into the scientific realm. I am certain that his work will ultimately have an impact on the "pure" sciences.

The Big Bang of God's Creation from the center of a singularity gave evolution to the universe, including us to be. So here we are as we are, because we were as we are, not far from the center of a unity.

—The Author

When you relate to your own center, you initiate a process of conscious development which leads to oneness and wholeness. You no longer see yourself as an isolated point on the periphery, but One in the center.

—Carl Jung (1875–1961)

What the center brings must obviously be that which remains to the end and was there from eternity. Nature has neither core nor outer rind, being all things at once. It's yourself you should scrutinize to see whether you're center or periphery.

—Goethe (1749–1832)

Our brains' answer seems to be about getting to the center of our unity, or maybe there is another way to say it.

—The Author

Introduction

This is an account of an experience in my life and what that experience has meant to me and may mean to you. It is an experience that varies as people vary, related to our most prevailing human condition and basic force. It is about a revolutionary idea that goes to our very core and has always been with us, but has been secret for lack of knowledge and understanding. It will be part of our future one way or another, knowingly or secretly. Are you ready for such an idea?

This book is an attempt toward an explanation of what our slowly evolved reflective consciousness has done to us and for us. It is a reconsideration of our long misunderstood metaphors of what has been happening deep within, somewhere and somehow within our brains. It is an attempt to suggest a clue toward creating an overall framework in the neurosciences and other areas. Even without a completely satisfactory scientific basis for our speculations, we need to get less skeptical and anxious about what has been called, among other things, our "soul center." The process we need to make us whole human beings gives meaning to our lives from the inside out, with some initial help from the outside in. For this reason, a variety of outside information is helpful, including perhaps the five chapters of this book:

Chapter 1 — *When* — In our maturity, something happens inside to interact with consciousness, causing a common experience unique to being human.

Chapter 2 — *Where* — Specific processes occur within the brain that need new words to assist understanding the experience.

Chapter 3 — *What* — Representations and derivatives of the experience are culturally expressed in great diversity.

Chapter 4 — *How* — Most people think of the experience as "religious."

Chapter 5 — *Why* — This experience happens because we and our brains are ready.

A well-known metaphor expressing how we became aware of ourselves or how we became human was set in a place located not far to the west, called Eden. It is an image of a circular garden with rivers extending in four directions from a center where there is a beautiful fruit tree. The underlying basis of this image and of thousands like it, and how we would not exist without them, is the subject of the following chapters. If you look carefully at this metaphor, you may see the leaves in the garden shimmering in the sunlight, and hear the sound of water and soft music. Somewhere nearby, a man and woman are talking about delicious fruit. They had been talking earlier of ancient times, how the snake in the garden represented becoming conscious of ourselves, and how the tree at the center and its fruit gave that knowledge. She goes closer to where he is sitting and presses against him. He buries his nose in her stomach, reaching around and raising her up, whispering, "Where is your snake friend?"

Yes, we should be thankful to all of those who bring us nourishing fruit from the tree at the center of their garden.

Chapter 1: The Neurostatic Experience

A Personal Reflection and Inquiry

This book is written for the primary purpose of sharing and explaining what I now refer to as my Neurostatic experience, which happened more than forty years ago, when I was twenty-four. I have since come to realize that it was an experience that many people have had, although in their own unique ways. Some would consider it a religious experience, which I feel is a limited reference. I have thought about this experience a great deal, why it happened and what it may mean, how common it is, and how it may give expression to our spiritual endeavors. In any event, I believe that this experience has a basis in physical reality, which I would guess is the result of our longtime selection and adaptation, allowing for self-consciousness. What is more certain to me is that the experience provides an empirical basis of what is generally known as the encompassing or larger self, or any metaphor that might be applied to the idea of this psychobiological transformation. It would seem that the process that gives rise to this experience may be important enough by itself neurologically to encourage research and a determination of how it works. Until then, we will continue not to know much more than the rehashed stories of conflicting truths of thc unknown happening inside us.

There have been times in the past when we became aware that we were not the center of everything. When new awareness removed us from a center, it was not generally acknowledged, although it was always acknowledged by some. Thinking of ourselves as the center of everything, including the universe, probably began naturally very early. It is an approach to life that has extended up to the present day. We still think we are the special center of God's concerns, but actually God is in our brains, which may be our new center. Yet, God is not a program, a group, a function of culture, or a way for social adherence. God does not come to you from the outside or inside of someone else's brain in the past, present, or future. We can know that the process of God and the meaning of ourselves come from how our own brains work.

It seems to me that our recent coming to worldwide systems of communication and dominion is showing a lack of meaning except on a local basis. This will not be resolved by a composite of tolerance for the world religions or massive new religions or ideologies. We have on Earth today about 2,000 languages and at least 150 religions with variations of gods. Continuing strife and suffering as a result of local exclusiveness may be our only response in the foreseeable future, unless there is enhanced awareness from increased common knowledge not yet known. In that regard, we should attempt to know more of how the brain works to bring ourselves to ourselves for our humanness and what becomes our spirituality. This process could then be expanded to a new understanding of human nature in general. We might start with the hypothesis that this experience has a neurophysiological foundation. Searching for our greater selves is something that many brilliant people have worked over in some form, and still do. That is reason enough by itself for venturing a serious attempt to include such searches within the realm of scientific review. For that, there may be a hint here to help with what to look for and how to proceed.

John Dewey, the influential American philosopher, contended that "a very humble experience is capable of generating and carrying any amount of theory, but a theory apart from experience cannot be grasped even as a theory. An ounce of experience is better than a ton of theory simply because it is only in experience that any theory has vital and verifiable significance."[1] My own conclusions come from direct experience and observation. I am posing an hypothesis that reinterprets the basis of the centuries-old spiritual, religious, or enlightened experiences in a new form that can be determined factually.

A secondary purpose of this book is to invite persons with similar experiences, or any other interested parties, to send in their comments or suggestions. I am interested in your experience or the experience of someone you know. At the present time, experience is the main exhibit of evidence.

Neurostasis, or What Some Would Call God

We have evolved over the ages toward self-identification, or I-ness. This natural brain evolution has caused a necessary postponement of overall brain development until the I-ness becomes sufficiently established. When that happens, we will experience at some point in our maturity a completeness with realizations of what some might call our larger self, wholeness of life, or God.

There have been a variety of names for this experience in different times and places: God, satori, nirvana, and so on. Since I wish to emphasize the combined physiological and psychological aspects of the experience, I would like to coin a new name for it. I call this process of making us whole human beings, or of achieving completeness within ourselves, "Neurostasis." The word is taken from *neuro* for "nerve," which refers to the total brain and spinal cord, and *stasis*, which refers to any regulating, stabilizing, or controlling center, or anything that checks, balances, or equates. The combination, *Neurostasis*, indicates a neurological approach to what has heretofore been considered from a religious approach with religious terminology that only confuses the issues.

Neurostasis occurs in at least three stages:

1. Types of stress eventually trigger within the brain, mediating neurochemicals or neurohormones.

2. The neurochemicals cause an abrupt electrochemical, permanent integrating synthesis of brain functions that previously had been held in check or had remained undeveloped.

3. This synthesis results in unity images being relayed to consciousness forcefully and vividly, from which a more encompassing personality is formed with a new sense of life.

These three stages involve more than simple electrochemical events. Human beings have been striving to have such experiences for thousands of years. In fact, without such experiences there would be no humans.

Neurostasis and the Gate of the Soul

It is not yet known precisely what part of the ancient core of our subcortical brain yields the Neurostatic experience. Nevertheless, this transformation of ourselves opens the gate of our soul. It gives us a profound sense of unity and a new view of life. It may be related to homeostasis in other forms. It may also be related to sleeping and dreaming, since people often have dreams of Neurostatic images. I know from my own experience and from the historical indications that there is without a doubt a neurophysiological facility and process that cause the Neurostatic completion of ourselves. Of the many questions in the brain sciences, one could add the following: what happens within what part of the brain to bring to our self-consciousness a vivid sense of unity or completion?

Whether you view Neurostasis scientifically, spiritually, or practically, our lives seem to follow a particular sequence:

1. When we are born, our brains have their original wholeness with minimal consciousness, mostly unconsciousness.

2. As we grow, so does our consciousness, out of which evolve the beginnings of self-consciousness. We become independent persons, with I-ness, separate from others, the world, and seemingly nature in general.

3. As we continue to grow from childhood, this development reinforces those elements within our brains that are related to self-awareness, instead of maintaining our brains' natural unifying processes. We proceed to become unwhole to assure that we become self-conscious, self-determining persons of free will and responsibility of action.

4. This neurological disparity, in effect a one-sided development, becomes more prominent in adolescence. During this time of maturation, however, the brain's disposition to re-

turn to its original wholeness or unity also begins to increase.

5. As we come into adulthood, with our separate I-ness sufficiently established, we become receptive to our wholeness or completeness. When that happens, it is normal for certain processes within the brain, goaded by self-consciousness, to bring to consciousness an experience of unifying images. This gives us a profound sense of unity—of being part of everything—with new realizations about life. This experience can happen earlier or later in life, depending on conditions within the person and possible diversions. We may come to it unknowingly in old age.

6. There is a natural inclination to avoid this intimate unknown. Neurostasis is commonly postponed with intellectual pursuits and the drives for work, marriage, and family. It is often taken care of indirectly by social and religious institutions and other groups that impose the use of various types of unity symbols that are related to the innate process of Neurostasis.

The Background of the Experience

When we are born, we start with wholeness to become unwhole. In this process of becoming ever more incomplete, we occupy almost a fourth of our lives growing up and becoming sufficiently self-conscious to operate in the world with confidence. In the past, it was helpful to have continuing religious or cultural conditioning to maintain that confidence. Without that confidence, we will at some point be in a blind search to make ourselves complete. The search is an unknown and can continue for a lifetime, during which we can become mellow, brittle, or lost, or we can find our original wholeness.

Following is a list of some of my youthful experiences from ages four to twenty-four. Although they may not seem unusual, this list does provide an indication of progressing from wholeness to unwholeness and back to wholeness.

1. Where Do We Come from, and Where Do We Go? I remember myself as a small boy sitting at the bottom of the stairway to heaven. It had marble steps and a golden handrail extending into the mist. I had been told that my oldest sister, who was ten, had gone to heaven. The stairway extended to the second floor of the hospital where she died after being hit by a car. Going to heaven was important. What can little boys of four know about heaven, of where and what it is? Perhaps little boys are still partially in heaven.

2. We Are Here with Life. One of the most exciting and mysterious events that I recall was waiting for eggs to hatch. In my family's hatchery, rack after rack of eggs piled to the ceiling were rolled into large incubators. Later, the racks were rolled out, filling my senses with hundreds of yellow and white crescendo-chirping chicks.

3. Socialization. Parents are persistent. First, I had to take piano lessons. At the age of five, I had to give two solo performances, one at church and one at school. Then they decided that I might like trumpet lessons better. Soon those were changed to drum lessons. Those were better, but they included a nonstop roll through the entire "Star Spangled Banner," and I couldn't keep up. All my brothers and sisters played the piano or some other instrument very well. I was the only holdout.

4. Going to the Center. There is water at the center of the Earth. In an area some distance beyond our family garden, there were large piles of dirt that seemed like mountains. That was where we built roads and towns for our toy cars and trucks. Between the mountains, there were old boards where you could toss rocks that disappeared. Crawling out on the boards and feeling the cool air coming up, we could drop rocks between the boards. It was a long time before a faint splash could be heard. After several tests, we decided that the distance was about to the center of the Earth. A year or so later, my parents had construction workers remove the boards, exposing a hole eight feet wide and a hundred feet deep. Then the men installed a windlass to lower and raise themselves as they lined the well with concrete. I took half a dozen rides into that deep center where there was water and darker deep beyond. When the men finished the construction, they lowered a pump to the bottom, and then a large pressure tank. I was watching with everyone else when the tank quietly slipped its chains and fell to the center of the Earth. While we held our breath, a weak voice down in the darkness finally said, "I'm okay." When he came up to the surface, we could see that the buttons and one pocket were missing from his denim jacket. Today, that well is the town's water supply.

5. The Power Around Us. I was born in the small town of Gove, in western Kansas. My early life was surrounded by the Great Depression of the 1930s. I lived through drought and dust storms that could be seen coming on the horizon from miles away, epidemics that killed livestock by the truckload, and grasshoppers darkening the skies and destroying crops on a vast scale. I watched tornadoes approaching, danced in lightning storms, and teased rattlesnakes. While growing up, all I had to do to feel the unimaginable power around me everywhere was to sleep out on the barn roof during hot summer nights in the arms of the Milky Way Galaxy, besieged by the massive extravagance of stars. One night, all the local people, including me, formed a human barricade on one side of town. We used car headlights to see what we were doing as we clubbed a mass migration of rabbits into taking a detour around the town.[2]

6. Adolescent Education. When World War II started, I was just eleven. We were gathered in one of the larger classrooms to listen to the radio as Roosevelt asked the Congress to declare war. Right after that, we moved to Dodge City, a larger town not far from Gove, where I lived through this strange time of everything saturated with war.

When I was fifteen, I read about the atomic bomb being dropped on Hiroshima. It seemed obvious that there would be no more war, since it would be suicidal for everyone. On the other hand, I felt cheated that the war was over before I could get into it. Being a teenager was not easy for me, but I did manage to finish Dodge City High and go on to college.

7. The Beginning Search. It was during my junior year in college that I happened to read an article by Lewis Mumford about the good life. Suddenly realizing that I had a lot of catching up to do, I became a bookaholic with a deep hunger for knowledge. I also wanted to get out of Dodge City, so at twenty I went west on the Oregon Trail.

8. The Scientific Method of What Can Be Done Will Be Done. The scientific method is predicated on testing hypotheses and theories of the material world of the senses. During summer breaks at college, one of my many jobs was to help remove trees from a farm at a place called Eight Dollar Mountain. It was said that someone had worn out a pair of eight-dollar shoes walking around it. My co-workers were an odd bunch—including the boss, who had a trunk full of papers from lawsuits in which she had been involved. The fat cook, who drove a big Cadillac and smoked huge cigars, advised me that to be an artist it was necessary to take drugs. There was also a mountain man who would axe a tree and tell funny stories with a hill-billy accent.

Then there was the old-timer who gave his Social Security checks to the boss so she would take care of him. Among his books was an old beat-up copy of the treatise that was part of the scientific revolution of almost four hundred years ago: the *Discourse on Method* by René Descartes. He has long been discounted because of his hypothesis that the brain's pineal gland is where the soul did its magic. He contended that the gland was a unity, not divided like most of the brain. Descartes's famous dictum is still around, "I think, therefore I am." I am too—especially as I think of the old-timer sitting on the porch swing, looking into the distance.

9. Compulsive Seeking. The lettering above the library doorway on campus was typical of short quotations seen on older public buildings: "You shall know the truth, and the truth shall make you free." I would go up into the stacks of the library and flip pages to accept or reject books in a random way. I lived for almost two years in those stacks, devouring books with a compulsion to catch up, to find the answer, to get free.

10. What Is This? When I was twenty-four, I walked one sunny midday through a backyard garden into an inside stairway to my room. I was standing next to the bed when what I sometimes call my wide-awake dream occurred. I hadn't drunk any alcohol, or taken any drugs, or been deprived of sleep. The dream may have come as a result of my two years of concentration, trying to determine what life was all about. For some time, I had been conducting an experiment on myself to find the answer to this question without relying on anyone else. As I stood there, I saw three-dimensional geometric configurations of overwhelming energy, light, and motion come together into an expanding circular radiance.

As a result of this experience, I had a feeling of complete reconciliation with myself, and I no longer had any need for answers to unanswerable questions. My whole life since that moment has been connected to that experience.

My Experience of Neurostasis

The following description provides evidence by direct empirical experience that the Neurostatic process happens. In this process, the brain first creates unity images. This is followed by the beginning of a changed awareness or consciousness. People who have had such experiences tend to write about the second phase, to the exclusion of the first.

It is difficult to describe such experiences in words. My description may not convey the strong effect the experience had on me, but I can assure you that I was transfixed. I didn't question or evaluate the images. In fact, I didn't *think* at all. I simply felt fresh and relaxed. I had no sense of time passing, but I would guess that the whole experience lasted no more than two minutes. I would also guess that my own Neurostatic experience would not be exactly like anyone else's. Like fingerprints, no two are ever identical. The only thing that all Neurostatic experiences have in common appears to be the centering or unifying effect with light. During Neurostatic experiences, our brains formulate unity. Although my Neurostatic experience was simultaneous and timeless, I will attempt to describe it as having a beginning, middle and end.

Beginning. As I stood beside my bed, I suddenly had the feeling that something was about to happen. Immediately, an image of a circular shape came toward me very fast on an arc from the right. Then an identical form came toward me from the left and merged with the first. My consciousness was completely taken over by the image. Churning with light and energy, the round shape developed a pulsing diagonal line across it. Then a diagonal line with a stepped or saw-tooth edge formed across the image in the opposite direction. The intersecting diagonals formed an x across the round shape, dividing it into quadrants. The diagonals then interchanged with each other until they merged with great force and energy, rotating the x into a plus sign (+). Then the lines faded away, leaving an energized area at the center of the circular shape. I had a subtle sensation of meshing.

Middle. Developing more energy and power, the circle evolved into a three-dimensional sphere with a band or indentation at its equator. The sphere pulsated with power and with light that was escaping through hundreds of holes, as if a monstrous furnace or small sun were burning inside. I had the feeling that the sphere was turning into a kind of life force.

End. The light emanating from the sphere became even brighter. Gradually, the sphere evolved into an overwhelming moving concentric pattern of bright colors. It became larger and brighter, extending outward and upward, filling everything with radiance. I became enveloped in the center of it, and it disappeared like a bubble.

Afterward. I stood there, accepting the experience without hesitation or question. It had not been unpleasant, particularly toward the end. I knew something unusual and extraordinary had happened, and I had an overall feeling of amazement. After a short while, I went for a walk and found a new world.

Years later, as I was reading the collected works of Carl Jung, whose writings tend to substantiate my own views, I thought of my Neurostatic experience when I came across the following passage:

> It is easy to see how the severe pattern imposed by a circular image of this kind compensates the psychic state—namely, through the construction of a central point to which everything is related, or by a concentric arrangement.... This is evidently an attempt at self-healing on the part of nature, which does not spring from conscious reflection but from an instinctive impulse. Here, as comparative research has shown, a fundamental schema is made use of, an archetype which, so to speak, occurs everywhere and by no means owes its individual existence to tradition.... Indeed, it could even be called the archetype of wholeness.... Because of this significance, the "quaternity of one" is the schema for all images of God.[3]

More recently, as I was reading a book about Hindu religion, I came across an image that reminded me of the shape in the beginning phase of my Neurostatic experience (see Figure 1).[4] The Hindu symbol of an undulating snake and a bamboo stick intersecting on a circular background has the same underlying structure as a part of my Neurostatic images. Very likely, this Hindu arrangement is derived from a Neurostatic experience that someone had a long time ago. According to the author of the book, the symbol appears on an ancient Hindu talisman, and is the sign of an initiate—that is, someone who is being introduced to knowledge. The circular shape represents the infinite universe, with the serpent as the creative energy life force or, in humans, consciousness. The seven joints of the bamboo stick represent chakras, or energy centers.

Affects of the Images

Immediately after the experience of the images, and during and after taking a walk, I felt that pieces of a puzzle were coming together. A few of those that I recall were:

> • The total experience was characterized by an overriding realization that, however briefly, I had a feeling of complete unity—that nothing exists apart from the whole. I felt that I was in and of everything, with a special affinity with all living things.
>
> • I came to know that there is an essence that is in everything—that everything is made from the same thing, from the greatest to the smallest, everywhere.

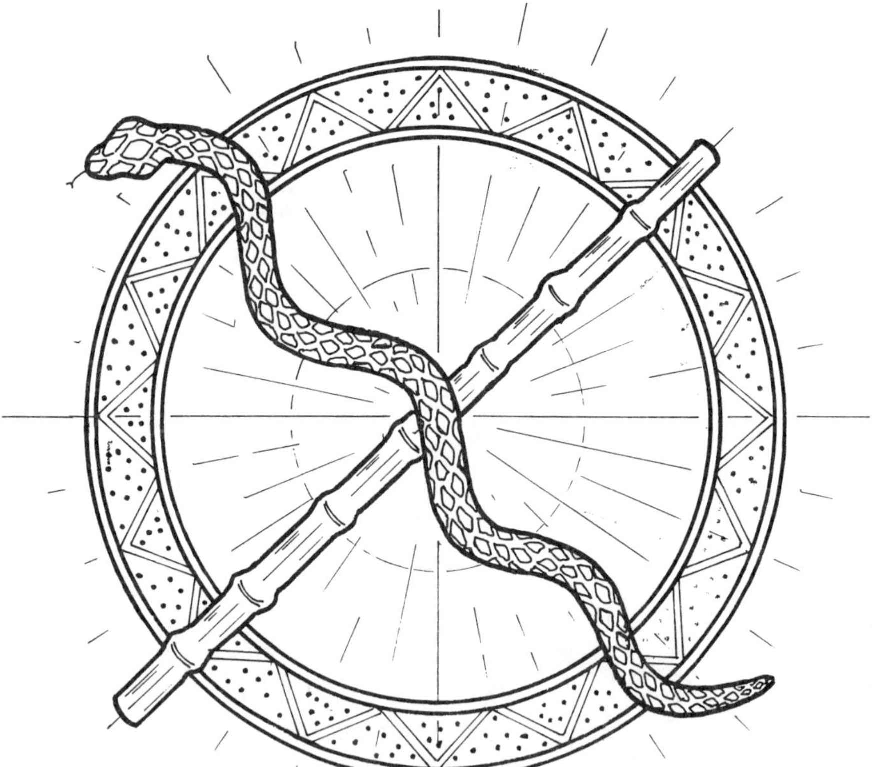

Figure 1:
Hindu Symbol

• I knew that the main purpose of life is to enjoy it in all ways, and to take things as they are, whatever they are.

• At the time, I would readily have sacrificed my life to save another person, if that had been necessary. I felt that we are all in this existence together.

• When I took a walk after my experience, I met a cat and felt intensely how connected we were. We were from the same mix and the same involvement.

• Material things no longer mattered to me. I completely trusted everything. Everyone is equal and unique.

• I am my own answer and my own meaning.

• We humans are not separate from nature, we *are* nature. Everything we are is in and of this Earth. There are no exceptions.

Current Afterthoughts

In thinking back today about my experience, I realize that the images and the aftereffects were not the source or instigator of my changed consciousness of unity. That was caused by fundamental underlying changes in my brain. The Neurostatic process gives consciousness, through images, a new unified self-identity that was not there before.

As the Neurostatic experience occurs, whatever is causing it is in control. To me the experience was completely unexpected and involuntary. My vision was totally taken over, both inwardly and outwardly. My normal mental activities were suspended, yet my awareness remained clear. During the experience, I had no self-consciousness, or I-ness. As a result, I did not try to do or not do anything. I did not think of myself. I did not create labels or make judgments. My senses all seemed to be working normally. The experience was like an addition to or expansion of myself, not a replacement of anything. I could only analyze the experience after it had happened.

Although this brain reorganizing process has been around for as long as we have been human, it is widely misunderstood because its neurophysiological components have not yet been determined. The process is natural and normal, and not some type of brain malfunction. The experience is not a form of trance in which one feels separate from regular sensory input. Neither is it an hallucination or illusion based on false or distorted perceptions. It is not caused by suggestion or hypnosis. One's awareness is not restricted, and one's self-image is preserved and expanded. There is no sense of separation between oneself and the experience.

There are numerous experiences that, in one way or another, resemble the Neurostatic experience but are nevertheless different from it. These include various conscious states caused by drugs, mental illness, some spiritual visions, and deprivation of sleep, food, or sensory stimulation. They all, however, differ from the Neurostatic experience in that in all of them one's I-ness or self-reference remains as a participant, and consciousness is reduced.

Can the Experience Be Described?

Obviously, the above description of my Neurostatic experience does not provide extensive detail. I have concluded that such experiences cannot be completely or satisfactorily described. The Neurostatic experience seems to be a process in which self-reference is minimized and the ability to analyze is severely restricted. The images of the experience are dynamic, with considerable light, energy, and emotional intensiveness that cannot be duplicated. The experience is all the more difficult to describe because it is an unexpected one-time event in our lives.

These limitations may be the reason that these experiences are typically communicated or represented in an indirect fashion with metaphors and symbols and are so overwhelming and mysterious that they are thought of as spiritual or religious. It is understandable, with these limitations, why there are not more descriptions of the actual experience of the Neurostatic images, rather than descriptions of how people felt *after* their Neurostatic experience was over. Jung speaks of this difficulty in the following passage:

> The existence of a transcendental reality is indeed evident in itself, but it is uncommonly difficult for our consciousness to construct intellectual models which would give a graphic description of the reality we have perceived. Our hypotheses are uncertain and groping, and nothing offers us the assurance that they may ultimately prove correct. That the world inside and outside ourselves rests on a transcendental background is as certain as our own existence.[5]

Neurostasis has been described in numerous ways in human history. In all its forms, however, it is a compensation for our development of self-consciousness and results in the experience of God in our brains. This in itself is sufficient to explain why the Neurostatic experience is so difficult to describe. When our consciousness and our physical being are ready for this experience, it comes.

Notes

[1]John Dewey, *Experience and Nature* (New York: Dover, 1958), p. 172.

[2]The Fick Museum in Oakley, Kansas, has photographs of a rabbit population estimated in the millions being clubbed to death during the 1930s.

[3]C. G. Jung, *The Archetypes and the Collective Unconscious* (New York: Pantheon, 1959), pp. 387–388.

[4]Mark Balfour, *Sign of the Serpent* (London: Prism Press, 1990), p. 27.

[5]C. G. Jung, *Mysterium Coniunctionis: An Inquiry into the Separation and Synthesis of Psychic Opposites in Alchemy* (New York: Pantheon, 1963), p. 551.

Chapter 2
Neurostasis—Inside Information

What Is Most Unique About Our Uniqueness?

There may come a time when you and I, like everyone else who has lived beneath the sky, will ask, "What does it mean?" The answer has always come from the sky or from someone to whom we gave the power of life and death, because we did not know our brains were working. Is the answer something from somewhere else, or is it in some way truly a reality of our own dear selves?

We should not be embarrassed or feel diminished that our brains and all that we are have evolved from the substances of the Earth and the universe in general, and those substances remain in essence a connection within our being and in all living things. Among those living things, only we with our self-consciousness have come to experience and be aware of these ties as inside information. The proposition of Neurostasis shows that a specific thing has been happening to us for a long time. It is a natural part of us, a remarkable experience that has a neurophysiological basis. This is a unique function of what our brains do. We humans are special among all living things, in that we have evolved additionally with self-consciousness, a lopsided development that is stabilized by an experience that appears to lead to our spiritual and religious endeavors. It is now no longer necessary, as in the past, to refer to this just as a spiritual phenomenon of experiencing God. We have to understand the unknown part of us, and this book offers a piece of the puzzle—a reality within our brains that we need to know more about.

I began writing this book by jotting down my thoughts about my own Neurostatic experience years ago. It seemed unusual then, and still does, since I am old enough now to know what effect it has had on my life. In attempting to write about that experience, I invite others to do the same, because we will eventually have to confront what this is and get wiser about the functions and processes of our brains, which give us ourselves. Whatever our Earth and the universe are, all of us are in this existence together, and we all have a natural ability to experience that existence in a very real way—a panhuman experience of factual happening beyond our I-ness.

My Neurostatic experience, described in Chapter 1, became a catalyst for the idea that we can have a profound experience resulting from an interaction between our brains and our consciousness. People often refer to this interaction as an experience of God. Although Neurostasis is a simple idea that may seem unlikely, its greater problem is the difficulty of expressing or explaining it. There is not a common language for it, and we do not yet know how the brain does it. I will poke around at this simple idea to see if I can bring it to life, which will require using some familiar terms.

The Neurostatic experience is known to many people in many areas of knowledge, both inside and outside scientific and religious organizations. To understand what I am talking about, think of traditional metaphoric expressions that attempt to describe the experience. There are many expressions to denote the experiencing of God, or a power beyond ourselves. These include being affected by forces of supernatural power, being saved or born again by a transformational experience, having a complete oneness between ourselves and the world, or receiving the light into our soul. These kinds of expressions are common in our lives. We have all heard of someone "getting" religion. For example, a pioneer diary from my wife's family has the following entry for a day in 1813:

> Mrs. Abernathy was the first to be converted a Methodist. Mr. Abernathy was so indignant that he forbade her attending the meetings. He was disappointed to find that the grown children were against him, saying that if Mother wants to attend meetings she ought to have the privilege. Later, Mr. Abernathy experienced religion at his home, about eleven o'clock at night. He shouted and praised the Lord so that he awakened all that were in the house. Both stayed with the church till their death.

A better record of this kind of experience in its many forms, extending back at least to shamanistic times, would make it obvious that something has been happening to us beyond what has been promoted by all the religious groups in history. We experience our brains through ourselves in an unusual way to cause these kinds of expressions to give meaning to our lives. A large part of most cultures, with their metaphors and symbolism, on a daily basis and across decades, is a striving toward the Neurostatic experience in the broadest sense.

There are three broad phases of being human that tend to meld together during our lives. They are why we have the capacity and need for religious or Neurostatic experience:

> 1. *Consciousness:* With our original wholeness as infants, we gradually become aware of the world around us. To some degree, all animals have this faculty. Consciousness begins with a neurophysiological process.
>
> 2. *Self-consciousness:* We extend our consciousness to include awareness of ourselves. This is the largest category of human activity. There are a number of names for this process, including "self-consciousness," "self-awareness," "self-identity," and "self-reference." It has also been referred to as "ego" or "I-ness." To have self-consciousness, one must

already have the potential for completeness-consciousness. Self-consciousness begins with a neurophysiological process.

3. *Completeness-consciousness:* We extend both consciousness and self-consciousness to include an awareness of the completeness of our original wholeness, while at the same time maintaining, preserving, and greatly expanding the sense of self. Completeness-consciousness is usually related to maturity and oriented to both our outside and inside worlds. It is sometimes called Enlightenment, Wisdom, Nirvana, Satori, Oneness, or Wholeness. Some people refer to it as becoming one with God, Allah, Yahweh, Mazda, or the Great Spirit. Completeness-consciousness begins with a neurophysiological process.

To Experience Our Brains Via Consciousness

In the final analysis, everything reduces to subjectivity, to our inside. There is no strict way of defining a separation or boundary between our subjectivity and what we regard as objective, or outside ourselves. To experience most things inside and outside ourselves is to be conscious of that experience. The brain's reflective consciousness often experiences many different functions and processes of both our inside and outside worlds. It is normal and not uncommon that we experience both worlds mixed together, not separated by self-consciousness. Just as we frown on people who talk to themselves, so we frown on the idea that all of us talk to ourselves. Nevertheless, we do all the time. We experience our brains via consciousness all the time. For example, our hormones activate various emotions and are activated by other emotions. This is all automatic, but we become conscious of the processes at some point.

We experience our brains via consciousness with learned and inherited behaviors of all kinds. We experience our brains via our consciousness by becoming aware of more of the cosmos than we can see. One of the most potent experiences that our brains provide is the emerging consciousness of images of what we have called God or many other names down through the ages. I am referring to those specific occasions when our consciousness experiences its own brain functioning in a way that could be called unification. We have such experiences because we have evolved with a kind of consciousness that is unique on this planet.

In the following pages, I will clarify how our brains briefly take control at some point in our lives, making us fully human by allowing us to become more aware of the world around us and to see ourselves as part of psychobiological whole. It is from the Neurostatic experience that we realize the meaning of life and how to conduct our lives. This book takes the old wisdom on this subject and applies it in an altogether new way. Extensive research will be needed to tease out the factual clues to explain how our brains actually facilitate the Neurostatic experience. At the present time, the processes, elements, or related neural correlates for this experience have not been established, although there have been some limited beginnings in the brain sciences.

If one were to go behind the human face mask to illustrate the brain within, the view would be what one sees in Figure 2, with bilateral symmetry extending throughout. Let us briefly review some of the functions of the different parts of the brain visible in the picture.

The *cortex* (tree bark) consists of the two hemispheres on the top of the brain. It provides for our capacity to be human. It is not what makes us function and operate, but it guides the *extent* to which we function and operate. The two cortical hemispheres are connected by and communicate with each other through the *corpus callosum*, which consists of more than two hundred million fibers. The duality of the cortex is connected with other dualities throughout the brain, including the following:

The *thalami* (bed chambers) are two main processors of all information of both the inside and the outside of ourselves. They can be thought of as relay or coordination facilities, perhaps as part of self-consciousness operations.

The *hypothalami* (below the bed chambers) are central structures between and below the two thalami. They

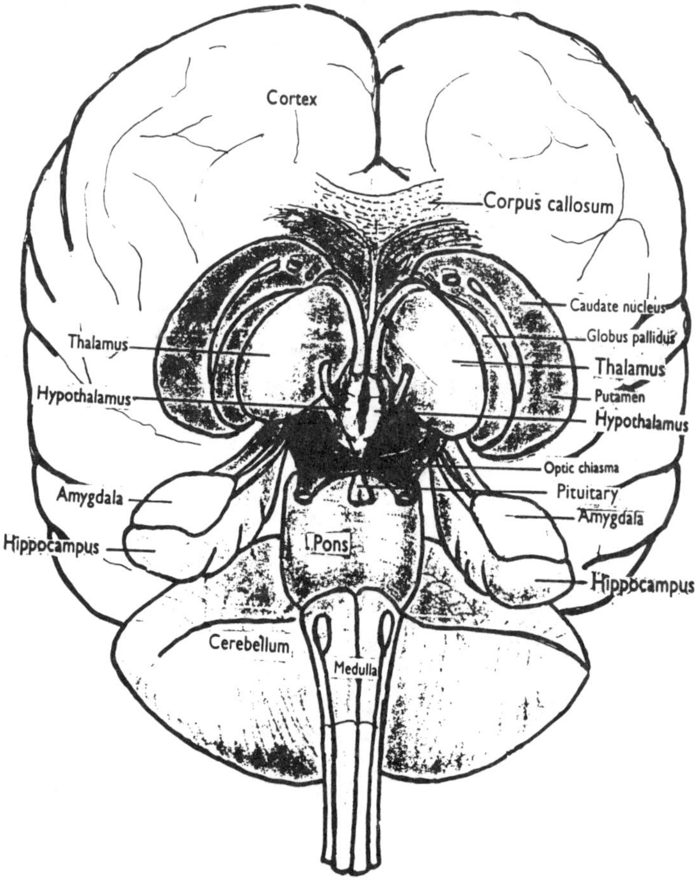

Figure 2:
Partial Front View of the Human Brain

control our emotions and regulate our sex drive, aggressiveness, pain and pleasure, and hunger and thirst. They provide homeostasis or balancing of our body's demands by giving direction to our hormonal processes.

The *pituitary gland* (waste carrier), suspended below the hypothalami, is the source of numerous types of hormones that act as controllers of other glands and tend to regulate behavior.

The *hippocampi* (horse sea monsters) are dual structures extending around the central area of the brain. They are directly involved in the storing and retrieval of most of our memories. Some experts believe that the hippocampi are related to our sense of self.

The *amygdalae* (almonds) are two small structures located toward the ends of the hippocampi. They are involved with primary emotions such as anger, fear, disgust, interest, joy, and sadness. They also seem to be critical sites for learning.

The *cerebellum* (little brain) is composed of two small hemispheres behind the brain stem. It is highly evolved in animals as well as humans, and allowed for the development of the human cortex while we were still swinging through the trees. The cerebellum regulates intent, coordination, direction, rate, movement, and balance. Remember this the next time you are watching an intense sports competition.

In the early 1900s, the River Neva in St. Petersburg, Russia, flooded during a spring thaw, leading to some laboratory dogs being terrified while trapped in their cages.

Their owner, Ivan Pavlov, noticed that they had unlearned everything he had taught them. This accident led him to theorize about the learning process. Later, his theories were unfortunately distorted to develop brainwashing techniques. On a more intellectual level, his ideas led to the dominance of behavioral psychology for over fifty years through the 1960s, first in American academia and subsequently in Europe. It was based on the concept that all human behavior reduces down to stimuli and responses, and that subjective phenomena and consciousness do not exist. This was a complete detour from the previous level of social consciousness represented in the ideas of William James and others.

Around the time that Pavlov was getting his dogs to salivate, the Spanish neurophysiologist Santiago Ramon y Cajal discovered the brain's synapses. Since then, scientists have been studying neurotransmitters and neurochemicals to learn how billions of brain cells or neurons communicate within our heads. For thousands of years, we have been looking for enlightenment or changed consciousness in drugs. Today, some people try to turn their heads into giant drugstores. We seem to have drugs and pills for everything, with ever more coming. Many of these are now being discovered by computers rather than by the usual laboratory methods.

In other research areas, we have developed tools such as the electron scanner, the nuclear microscope, and the laser microscope, which have been helpful in understanding the molecular and cellular plasticity of the brain. There is also gene and DNA research and the genome project to identify our replicators. In addition, we now have several devices, which will surely be improved upon, that allow us to see the brain in action on computer screens.

In the 1950s, Roger Sperry and others, separating the cortex areas to relieve epilepsy, unexpectedly found that the two sides of the cortex might have separate functions. This led to research and profound speculations about our left and right brains. Some people believe that we have two separate selves. Others believe that our two cortex areas are only contributors to the creation of one self, which has its more direct sources in the older biformed core areas of the brain.

Neurostasis and Our Evolved Brains: Six Questions

Several questions about Neurostasis suggest themselves.

First: Are human beings mysterious? Below the surface of the religious metaphors and symbols of every culture, there is something that they all share in common: the experience of the brain's evolutionary development and need for human completeness. All groups and organizations in history have devised metaphors and symbols to satisfy this need, and with that came the natural inclination to accept the unknown as mysterious. The mystery of life cannot be eliminated, nor would we want it to be, but I suspect the functions of our brains are no more mysterious than the functions of our whole bodies. We are just functioning in an ignorant way.

Why have we been told that our inside world does not belong to us, but to a power outside of ourselves to whom we should pray and worship? Getting right with ourselves is important. Being part of a community is essential for human beings, but the community is not essential for the Neurostatic power that is within ourselves. That power resides naturally in our brains with its own connections not sanctioned by anyone. The Neurostatic experience is the brain's way of giving us the answer to the meaning of life. From my own experience and what I have read and know about the experiences of others, Neurostasis only occurs once in a lifetime. Besides being unrepeatable, it comes unpredictably and unannounced. It is something we seek, often desperately, but we don't know how to make it happen. Nevertheless, when it does happen, it is totally understandable.

World history has largely been the organized symbolic and metaphoric reuse of someone's spontaneous Neurostatic experience—whether that person be named Zoroaster, Buddha, Jesus, Manes, Mohammed, or whatever. Invariably, this becomes the means and contrivance for collective authoritarian hierarchical adherence, either religious or political, or both. Religious or ideological conversion takes the individual's potential for Neurostasis and reshapes it in a collective mold. On the political stage, this is essentially a form of brainwashing.

The real human mystery is that from the time we are born we start the process of moving from unconscious wholeness to conscious unwholeness. That is, we begin complete and gradually become more and more incomplete. With the coming of adulthood, we finally strive to be complete again. We often accommodate to whatever group is available that will help us with this, but we are at a state of evolutionary consciousness where we can and should do it ourselves. This process of bringing forth our natural wholeness, or of experiencing God in our brains, does not diminish the mystery in and around us. The experience of Neurostasis enlarges and reinforces the mystery in the smallest to the largest life forms.

Second: Are we one brainminding whole entity? For the brain, there is no turn-on and no turn-off. The brain never stops. From its beginning to its ending, it is everything. The brain is always reaching outward and inward with activity or intentions we call "mind." This includes everything that is genetically determined, everything that operates the body, and, most important to us, everything that we learn and unlearn. Collectively, this has evolved outside ourselves into what we call culture, forming a kind of collective self-consciousness. It allows a totality of human expression, thought, and emotion outside our brains, since anatomically these things do not exist as such within our brains. There is nothing in our heads except physiological tissue of one sort or another.

No one can exist separate from his or her brain. Our consciousness, mental capacity, mind, soul, intelligence, and unconsciousness are not disembodied from the brain. All the forces of our brains are within our brains. The presumption of duality, such as creating a separation between brain and consciousness, or material and spiritual, derives from a lack of conditioning related to Neurostasis. The many forms of duality as separate entities are dispelled with the experience of Neurostasis.

Our brains work the way they do because of their long affair with evolution. For thousands or even millions of years, our brains have been running and operating without being told how, and they still do. Who was in control before we became conscious of ourselves?

The more we learn about our brains, the more impressed we will be with their complexity and capacity. The emotional evaluation of all our thoughts will also become more accepted. We could be living in dangerous times because of how dangerously ignorant we are of how our brains work. What we do know is that one of the main objects of brains and all living creatures is to preserve the conditions of life and keep it whole.

One of the most important attributes of our humanness is the degree to which we have come from the unknown, our unconsciousness. This is reflected in our own fossil past, which shows how we have physically distanced ourselves from what we have been and also from other animals.

Third: Are we organized to take care of ourselves? Our Earth is a vast organizing system. All of its organisms, including us, maintain systems of wholes that could not exist long without constant input and output of energy, substance, and information. Organic warm-blooded creatures, including us, have a remarkable self-maintaining brain-monitored mechanism called homeostasis, which maintains a balance of physical conditions with a sufficient amount of consciousness for us to live and grow. Beyond this, and even more remarkable, is Neurostasis, our own additionally developed self-maintaining natural process to maintain a stable self.

With the help of our emotions, our self-consciousness causes us at some time to feel incomplete in a world of opposites, polarities, and complementarities. Perhaps God made a mistake, or at least a design flaw, with all the dominant duality of either/or thinking and the difficulty of making choices. These choices have been troublesome to us ever since, because of the way our brains developed with their reflective consciousness and increasing knowledge. The human animal, when acquiring more consciousness than other animals, made adjustments in the brain for the increasing self-knowledge in conjunction with the loss of unconsciousness. We experience the world through opposites because our kind of consciousness has divided the world. It may be our purpose in life to reunify ourselves so we can experience the world as whole again.

Although we are organized to take care of ourselves,

it seems that God or our own evolution has not provided a good understanding of how the process or brain adjustment works or given us a clear way to explain it to others. The religions of the West and the East have different metaphors for the brain's adjustment to self-knowledge. In the West, one has an exchange with a power beyond oneself. In the East, one becomes enlightened. Human history indicates that we have been metaphorically confused, since there has never been agreement about what we are attempting to explain or represent. If we are going to take better care of our total selves, we will have to discover where and how the meaning of existence comes to us. Knowing this is basic to our being and survival.

Fourth: Are we going to talk about our metaphors? When people have a Neurostatic experience, they almost always describe it in metaphoric terms. The usual function of a metaphor is to describe something indirectly or by analogy when direct description is difficult or impossible. The more abstract features of human experience are best grasped in terms of broad conceptual metaphors. We could not have language without metaphor. Describing a tree without referring to anything else is not easy, but more difficult is describing an inner experience with the best of metaphors. For example, consider the phrase "father who art in heaven." The "father" is a male parent who represents God, and "heaven" is God's home in the sky. Alternatively, one might say, "God is an infinite sphere whose center is everywhere and circumference nowhere." Is this metaphor any better or any worse than the other?

With most traditional metaphors of our inner life, we project part of ourselves onto the outside world, making it separate from the organic realm of our bodies and brains. For example, the "Holy Ghost" is a metaphor that is disembodied from us, but will come and "visit" us. Clearly, this is something of our inner workings. Some people have used the metaphor of the machine to describe the brain. In its most recent incarnation, this metaphor has taken the form of the computer. Some enthusiasts believe that computers will eventually have a human-like consciousness that requires emotion. If so, perhaps such machines will have an experience of God, with more metaphors.

For millennia, we have used all kinds of unrestrained metaphors to represent our insides. All the while, however, we have ignored what our brains have been doing to us and for us. When it comes to Neurostasis, we may be greatly misunderstanding all the traditional metaphors related to it. New metaphors will be needed when it is finally determined that "religious experiences" are our brains' extraordinary responses to how we have evolved over time.

Peter Atkins, a physicist at Oxford University, contends "that the world has the same structures as mathematics or that they are the same. That the deep structure of the brain may be in resonance with the deep structure of the universe."[1] This "deep structure" may represent the process that allows for Neurostasis. The universe, as expressed by the existence and evolution of Earth, has forces of deep structure through everything. Perhaps our brains, with their relatively advanced awareness, occasionally reflect those forces. In this metaphor, there are mathematical formulas or patterns to provide a connection between us and the cosmos, the ultimate. These patterns exist in all mathematics, from Pythagoras to Einstein. Numbers have always been part of our consciousness and have always been metaphors. Current research indicates that humans used numbers long before they had speech.

Another cosmic metaphor has been suggested by biochemist Rupert Sheldrake, who deals with "morphic fields" and "morphic resonance":

> A morphic field is within and around a self-organizing system to organize its characteristic structure and pattern of activity..., which contains an inherent memory transmitted from previous similar systems by morphic resonance. Morphic resonance involves the transmission of formative influences through time and space.[2]

Sheldrake indicates that an entirely new, evolutionary conception of matter and field is coming into being in all the sciences. In general, the cosmos now seems more like a growing and developing organism than an eternal machine. In this context, Sheldrake suggests that habits of nature may be more natural than immutable laws. "Morphic fields," he says, "like the known fields of physics, are non-material regions of influence extending in space and continuing in time. They are localized in and around the systems they organize."[3] That is, each natural system has its own kind of field, and such fields shape all the different kinds of atoms, molecules, crystals, living organisms, societies, customs, and habits of brain activities. The process by which the past becomes the present within these morphic fields, Sheldrake calls "morphic resonance," which "involves the transmission of formative causal influences through both time and space. The memory within the morphic fields is cumulative, and that is why all sorts of things become increasingly habitual through repetition."[4] This may be why we perpetuate human attributes such as self-consciousness.

Sheldrake also speaks of "self-resonance" or "internal resonance":

> The most specific morphic resonance acting on a given organism will be that from its own past, because it is more similar to itself in the past than to any other organism. This self-resonance will therefore tend to stabilize and maintain organisms in their own characteristic form, as well as harmonizing the development of symmetrical structures within the same organism.[5]

Self-resonance may be the internal force that generates the Neurostatic images of unity and the resulting consciousness of wholeness. The resonance in and around our brains is that of our original wholeness before we were born. This is a wholeness that comes from a longtime force extending back in our evolutionary past. The morphic resonance of our brains—which I call Neurostatic activity and others call religious experience—stabilizes and maintains our brains' characteristic form of wholeness. This self-resonance harmonizes all the structures and functions within ourselves, including self-consciousness.

To resonate to the ultimate source of our inner lives, it is not necessary to develop mathematical theorems or to find patterns outside ourselves. There are other ways to do it. Our brains have many built-in capacities for dreaming, singing, humming, whistling, dancing, and making rhythm or other forms of resonance. Try one or more of these.

We need to talk more about our symbolic language and the meaning of our metaphors. Our long history of social gossip has stimulated our capacity for empathy, and ultimately has led us to ask ourselves profound questions about the meaning of life. The need for meaning has made us all self-aware, which has evolved into our outside memory, which we call culture.

We must always remember that in human communication there is always a part that is left unsaid. In fact, all of the communication can never be said, no matter how far you stretch it. As a result, we use metaphors and symbols to express the whole. How we have evolved with different kinds of wholeness has been shown by Julian Jaynes, who contends that, from the time of the development of language to about the seventh century B.C.E., people in various parts of the ancient world, including the Mediterranean, the Middle East, India, and China, were in effect divided into two parts operating bicamerally.[6] One part, called God, was an executive who gave directions in voices that were thought to come from the outside—much like voices heard today by schizophrenics, which often have a religious character. The other part was an ordinary person considerably less self-conscious than we are today:

> The presence of voices which had to be obeyed was the absolute prerequisite to the conscious state in which it is the self that is responsible and can debate within itself, can order and direct. In a sense, we had become our own gods.[7]

If what Jaynes says is valid, it may have been some time after the seventh century B.C.E. before there was adequate self-awareness to cause what we know as religious experiences, or what I call Neurostasis. People with a sufficient self-consciousness to have such experiences would have been considered extraordinary individuals and were likely the object of cult adoration. Later, the lives of these persons might be incorporated into a symbology to provide an indirect experience for a great many other people in social organizations, many of which still exist. Today, thanks to knowledge now available to us, humanity may be at the beginning of another transitional period, in which our level of self-awareness is quite adequate for us to complete ourselves. Finding "wholeness" or "God" can now be experienced by ordinary individuals directly for themselves without secondhand help from an intermediary or social organization.

Fifth: Are we going to get it right? There have been innumerable groups, large and small, in human history that have provided in some manner for the glory of God or gods to bring wholeness to their members. Most of these groups felt that their answers were eternally true, but history has shown that many of them were suited only to their time and place. However, their truths were variations of a truth from a more basic source, our brains. Humanity has always strived to be less unconscious, and in so doing, its truths have changed. This may always be so. As Jung commented:

> The unconsciousness wants to flow into consciousness in order to reach the light, but at the same time it continually thwarts itself, be-

> cause it would rather remain unconscious. That is to say, God wants to become man, but not quite.[8]

When we reach the light a little more, we will become individually more self-aware. Then we will begin to appreciate new things about old facts from around the world and down through history. From ancient times, at least as far back as the beginning of agriculture, many techniques have been devised to bring people into the mysteries of enlightenment. Religious and cultural disciplines had initiates participate in experiences that imparted secret wisdom and mysterious knowledge. It was, and still is, secret wisdom and mysteries, because it is not widely known how we relate to ourselves to experience ourselves. It was Aristotle, I think, who said that persons who were being initiated were not to learn anything but to experience something and be put in a certain condition. The secrets that the initiates experienced were inaccessible to outsiders.

We are fortunate that the human brain is not a closed system of fixed determinations as it is with other animals. Neither is it a slave to what it gets from the outside world. It is interactive, self-organizing, and capable of generating its own information. It has evolved to deal with both internal and external worlds. It would be less difficult for both worlds if we could understand what is happening in and between them by having a common language for both. Compared to the outer world, we know almost nothing of our inner world—that is, of how the brain works. The brains of all animals have selected the best way to react to their outside worlds and have developed consciousness accordingly. The human brain went a little further by selecting and adapting for more consciousness than other animals possess.

The most striking feature in the development of this greater consciousness is our sense of self or singleness of being. Nevertheless, the brain does not process one operation at a time but millions of simultaneous events. The individual senses that one being is having these experiences. This being changes somewhat from moment to moment and from day to day, but remains in essence the same self—a lifetime continuum of being. The self is an internal image created by nature's own workings, a natural representation formulated by the brain, completely removed from any conscious intention. Life as we know it is bound to individual carriers, each one of which is charged with an individual destiny and destination. This understanding alone makes some sense of life, although the self needs support from others for it to establish and maintain itself with the outer world.

For the first part of our journeys as carriers of life, we largely learn our I-ness in reaction to the surrounding environment and cultural context. We grow up, learn the rules, survive, and make an identification for ourselves as we attempt to separate from nature. As we approach our more complete biological maturity, usually in our late teens or early twenties, we begin to feel a need to know more of our secret inside, to reflect and search. It is then that we take a stand with the world to force answers to what our unknown original self means on one's own terms. The search culminates in a process whereby the brain naturally completes itself, giving to self-consciousness or I-ness a sense of our larger or more complete self. This is the wholeness that our I-ness needs to relate to, for us to be fully human. The process provides a subjective awareness of the source of our self-consciousness or I-ness. As Jung says:

> The self, like the unconscious, is *a priori* existent out of which the ego evolves. It is, so to speak, an unconscious prefiguration of the ego. It is not I who creates myself, rather I happen to myself.[9]

We have always organized to provide a symbolic program for the search for wholeness. This involves individuals submitting to a group's program, imposed from the outside. This makes those individuals a part of an organization. The experiences provided by all organizations and groups are all ways to show how you can experience

God, and thus become complete. It is now not enough for us to experience God through an organization; we also want to know *why* and *how* and *where in our brains* we experience God.

Sixth: Are we temporarily incomplete in order to become complete? When a child is very young, its brain is still intact as a whole, as with other animals. The last indications of no longer being whole in this world are the significant abilities both to talk and to remember. This is shown during the third and fourth years in children's art, when they do natural unity or wholeness drawings such as circles, concentric circles, and crosses or x's with centers. As a child grows, its inherited brain matrix, which only humans have, provides a growing separateness and individuality. With ongoing development of self-awareness, the child proceeds in subsequent years to drawings of people, houses, trees, and other representations of the outside world. While growing with this increasingly separate individuality, the child undergoes a natural corresponding disproportionate development of areas and processes of the brain about which little or nothing is known at the present time.

Our early brain development to adulthood allows for our growth to know who we are, to create an I. When our initial growth becomes adequate to this end, our bodies try to make us aware of what we left behind and of the need for additional growth, which our self-consciousness then attempts to provide. Perhaps for the rest of our lives, we have a continual unknown urge to somehow reflect ourselves to ourselves, in order to reestablish our original wholeness. Many people have found this in many ways. Socrates expressed it as "Know thyself." Thanks to our thousands of years in this effort, we have a need for a sense of completion toward a special kind of equilibrium, which is an expression of the biological process, simple or complicated as that may be.

We usually achieve this return to wholeness by being absorbed into an existing cultural group such as a religious, political, military, or similar organization. We have a natural, sometimes desperate drive to complete ourselves. But we also have a tendency to want to avoid completing ourselves by indulging in sex, family, work, or survival. Such avoidance can last a lifetime. Other distractions can include alcohol and drugs, even psychedelics, which may be helpful in some respects but not in the long run. Perhaps we are not so much avoiding our completion as not knowing what is happening to us. We blindly adhere to our conditioning and remain in any group that takes care of us. A large part of this is our need for community and bonding.

There are some people who will unconsciously strive to complete themselves at any cost. This striving has its own discipline, which goes wherever the striving goes. At times, such individuals may feel that they will either go crazy, kill themselves, or get through it. As Jung says:

> The attainment of wholeness requires one to stake one's whole being. Nothing less will do; there can be no easier conditions, no substitutes, no compromises.[10]

In 1902, William James similarly indicated that people become uneasy about something incomplete within themselves, but that there is a solution to the problem. "The uneasiness," he said, "is a sense that there is something wrong with us as we naturally stand. The solution is a sense that we are saved from this wrongness by making proper connection with the higher powers."[11] In other words, we are saved by trusting ourselves to find a greater understanding. Up to now, most scientific knowledge conditions us to be aware of the existence of the whole, but it cannot yet affirm or prove the existence of that whole.

Our Brain-Caused Unity Is the Experience of Neurostasis

The six questions above all relate to our being born complete, separating from that completeness, and then ultimately seeking to regain it. Those questions raise still other questions that will require additional research. For example:

- Are there different intensities of the Neurostatic experience? Could it also occur in a series of smaller, less intense experiences?

- Is there a way to grow to maturity without being part of, or conditioned by, a religious or similar group?

- Can we achieve a better understanding of the relationship between God in our brain (Neurostasis) and all that beyond us that we cannot comprehend?

- How possible is it to go through life with no more than me-ness?

- What have the changes been in Neurostasis, related to the evolution of consciousness? How do those changes relate to religious or cultural history?

- How do the different symbols and metaphors of different religious groups affect the type or quality of their Neurostatic experiences?

- Without knowing the brain's processes, can we act on the idea of Neurostasis?

- When the physical basis of Neurostatic processes becomes known and accepted, what will that mean to our concept of ourselves as humans, and how will that eventually affect society? What are the ramifications?

There could be and will be a great many more questions. As we mature, this process is something our brains need and want from the ongoing seeking of our self-consciousness. Until the brain's workings are better understood, we can proceed in an empirical way with the knowledge of our history and the testimony of those who have had the Neurostatic experience and a more open understanding of themselves.

During Neurostasis, besides ordering and orienting information, the brain integrates and unites experience in a predominantly affective manner that is beyond conscious will. Prolonged stress in a person's life is often resolved by an emotional completion or unification within the brain. When this happens, one becomes conscious of basic and fundamental images with very intense emotions. These images usually take the form of circular or spherical shapes with a centering effect. At the same time, there is an exuberance of light and energy. The images, which I call Neurostatic images, have the common motif of expressing completeness or wholeness. When the brain brings the images to consciousness to be experienced in some unity form, it causes a feeling of transformation with a direct understanding of ourselves. As Jung says:

> It can be expressed by roundness, the circle or sphere, or by the quaternity as another form of wholeness. I have called this wholeness that

> transcends consciousness the "self." The goal of the process is the synthesis of the self.[12]

At another point, Jung says about this:

> It is in the first place a purely natural process which may in some cases pursue its course without the knowledge or assistance of the individual, and can sometimes forcibly accomplish itself in the face of opposition. The meaning and purpose of the process is the realization, in all its aspects, of the personality originally hidden away in embryonic germ-plasm; the production and unfolding of the original, potential wholeness. The images used by the unconsciousness to this end are the same as those which mankind has always used to express wholeness, completeness, and perfection: symbols, as a rule, of the quaternity and the circle.[13]

Historically, these kinds of images and their subsequently derived symbolic interpretations have had universal distribution throughout traditions and societies up to the present time. These Neurostatic images have almost always come to consciousness as circular shapes, often radiant from a center, creating a process of complementary quarterly features with considerable light and encrgy. From these images come all the metaphors and symbols of completeness, unity, oneness, and wholeness throughout history. They have also been the schema for all the symbols of God. Erich Neumann says of such images:

> The uniting symbol is the highest form of synthesis, the most perfect product of the psyche's innate striving for wholeness and self-healing, which not only "makes whole" all conflict, provided that it is taken seriously and suffered to the end by turning it into a creative process, but also makes it the point of departure for a new expansion of the total personality.[14]

An important feature of these images that the brain creates is their symmetry, which is the natural innate expression of our completion, the Neurostatic process. Symmetry is natural at all levels of complexity of developing organisms. The structures and functions of our bodily organs, including our brains, are basically identical from one person to another. As our self-consciousness is completely dependent on the brain, presumably it will everywhere produce the same symmetrical forms. However, like snowflakes, no two of these forms are ever completely identical.

Approximately six months before I had the Neurostatic experience described in Chapter 1, I painted the picture seen below in Figure 3. On several occasions when I returned in the evening from the university campus, I became transfixed by a scene at a street intersection right in front of my house. There was a streetlight extending from a high pole, creating a radiance that shone through an autumn tree in the late evening twilight. One night, when I was at a friend's house, I painted the scene from memory. It seems to have been a prefiguration of my brain working for Neurostasis. I eventually entitled it "The Secret Where Four Streets Meet."

About twenty years after my Neurostatic experience, I made several attempts to capture the images I had seen, with only minimal success. Figure 4 reproduces a painting that attempts to capture an image from the middle part of the experience, as described in Chapter 1.

Since We Just Got Here, We Were Just Created

The next time you are out walking, take a look at a leaf and the unity of its bilateral symmetrical structure. Or examine the fruit from a tree you are about to eat. Or look at any organic object, and you will see growth from the inside-out. All of these demonstrate a force for balanced growth—which we can see in our own bodies. Millions and millions of years ago, at the start of life, unicellular embryos divided into two equal hemispherical cells. These cells then divided again to produce quar-

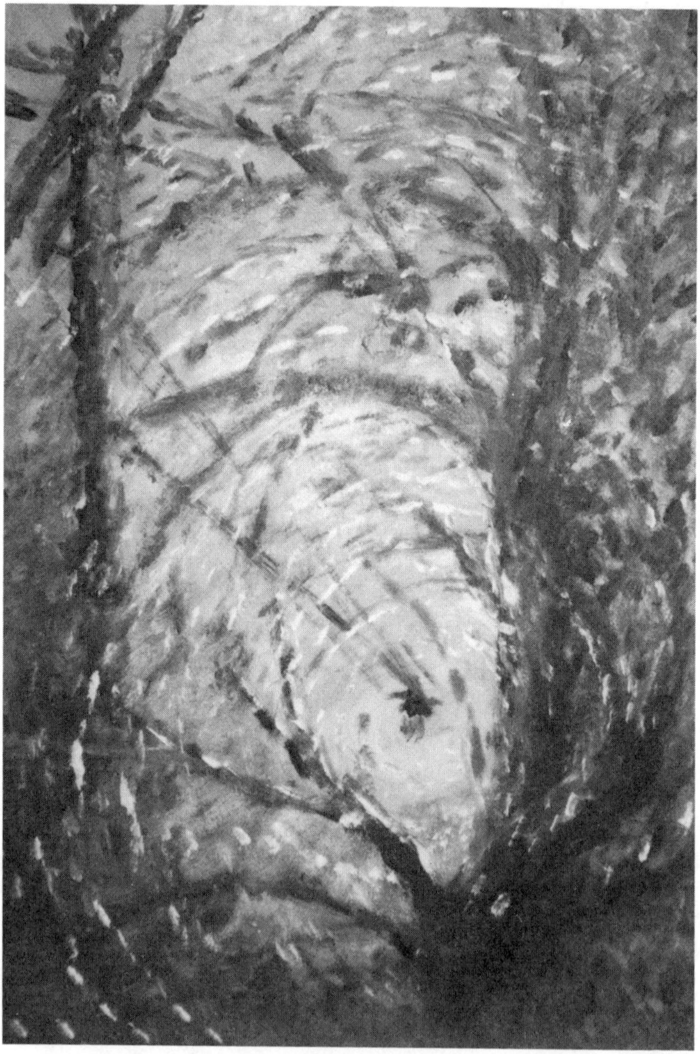

Figure 3:
"The Secret Where Four Streets Meet" (1953)
Painting by the author
(oil on paper, 16" w x 23" h)

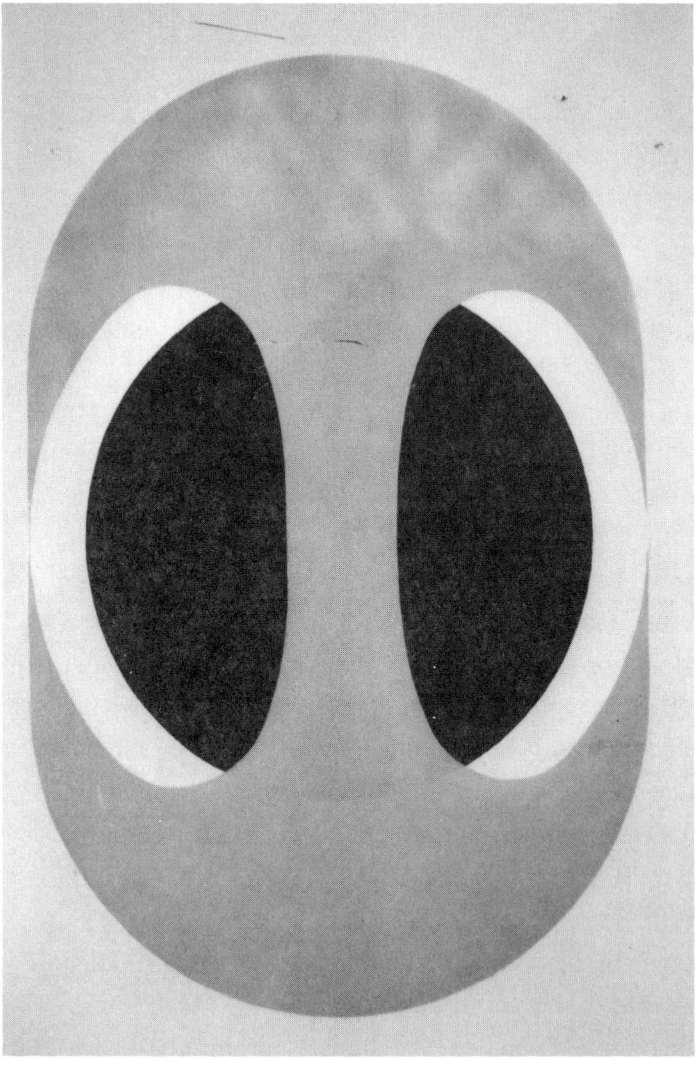

Figure 4:
"An Unsuccessful Attempt" (1973)
Painting by the author
(acrylic on hardboard, 6' w x 4' h)

ter spheres, and the process of symmetrical growth continued on.

Substantial parts of our body incorporate bilateral symmetry on our left and right sides. This is particularly true of the brain and spinal column. The brain is not one thing but two things joined at the center. It begins as a folding, becomes a neural tube with swellings at one end, and ultimately turns into a hindbrain, midbrain, and forebrain. This reflects the evolutionary development of three brains in stages, all with bilateral symmetry. Within this symmetry, brain processes are dual in all directions—up-down, side to side, crisscrossed, and looped. It works as a dynamic whole.

Millions of years of evolution have brought us to where we are today. You and I would not be here unless someone or something had been here before us. We and all other living creatures are part of the same basic plan. The presence of the past is very much with us. Our first distant relatives to have brains with components similar to ours were vertebrates extending back about five hundred million years. They included fishes, amphibians, reptiles, birds, and mammals, all characterized by a segmented spinal column and a distinct differentiated head. The brain that evolved that was most similar to ours began with our primate forefathers and foremothers forty to seventy million years ago. As Richard Leakey has suggested, "The first human species can best be described simply as bipedal apes."[15] Those ancestors of ours had a prehuman consciousness. About four million years ago, we developed a somewhat human appearance, but our brains were not yet what they are today. We walked and ran upright, as we do today, perhaps even better, but retained our primitive prehuman heads and brains. Our brains were about half their present size, and our self-awareness was comparably less. We lived mostly with the unity of nature in the world of Eden.

Early humans were able to judge, reason, solve problems, and perform most of the things we do now, except they had minimal self-awareness, I-ness, God, or reflections on culture. As with other animals, early humans did not need self-awareness to operate in the world. In the last ten thousand to a hundred thousand years, these protohumans significantly increased their consciousness, finally approaching the consciousness we have today. Thus, as humans we just got here. You could say we were just created.

Other animals, even other primates, are born with a brain nearer to its ultimate development than is the human brain at birth, which develops substantially after birth. A new human brain has less than a fourth of the weight of a fully developed adult brain. The young brain grows and forms while adapting to life to become independent and self-aware. This results in parts of the brain developing at different rates.

We are slowly and collectively learning a new story for ourselves, a more universal myth or metaphor: that life evolves as does everything. Our story should show that we now have an elaborated ancient brain resulting from millions of years of selection and adaptation to finally make it a brain of self-consciousness. It has taken a while, but now, after all the struggle, we finally have recognition. Soon, our consciousness will know that God is in our brains.

Antonio Damasio, the chairman of the Department of Neurology at the University of Iowa, stated that "the soul and the spirit, with all their dignity and human scale, are now complex and unique states of the organism."[16] Other researchers have started to probe exactly where in the brain experiences reside that I call Neurostatic.

For example, Paul MacLean of the National Institute of Health in Washington, D.C., a longtime researcher in the neurosciences, has stated that it is the limbic system of the brain, the area surrounding and above the brain stem and below the cortex, that gives us our sense of self and our sense of truth. "Without a co-functioning limbic system," he writes, "the neocortex lacks not only the requisite neural substrate for a sense of self, of reality and the memory of ongoing experience, but also a feeling of conviction as to what is true and false."[17] Locating our sense of self and truth in a particular region of the brain indicates that we are getting closer to the neurophysical features of Neurostasis, where our soul gate is.

Researchers at the Center for Brain and Cognition, at the University of California, San Diego, have determined that there are areas of the brain that may affect how intensely a person responds to religious beliefs. In experiments with patients with an unusual form of epilepsy who had previously reported mystical experiences as part of their seizures, it was determined that one effect of the experiments was the strengthening of the brain's involuntary response to religious words. Further studies may show which specific areas of the brain are involved with religious experiences.[18] The Director of the Center, V. S. Ramachandran, asks the question:

> Could it be that human beings have actually evolved specialized neural circuitry for the sole purpose of mediating religious experience? The human belief in the supernatural is so widespread in all societies all over the world, that it's tempting to ask whether the propensity for such beliefs might have a biological basis.[19]

Neurostasis is knowing where our center is. Finding where and how our center exists will provide a means to know how we evolved and why we were created the way we are. The ancient idea that we can seek and sometimes find the naturally occurring experience of Neurostasis, and biological attempts to determine the physical basis of Neurostasis, should not be viewed as threatening to either our spiritual heritage or our scientific traditions. The striving for knowledge in all forms will always be part of us. It would be easier to explain the Neurostatic experience if we all had a common vocabulary for our inner experiences, and if there were more neurophysiological facts about the functions of the brain.

Notes

[1]Peter Atkins, *Creation Revisited: The Origins of Space, Time and the Universe* (New York: W. H. Freeman, 1992), pp. 109 and 119.

[2]Rupert Sheldrake, *The Presence of the Past: Morphic Resonance and the Habits of Nature* (Rochester, Vt.: Park Street Press, 1988), p. 359.

[3]Sheldrake, *Presence of the Past*, p. xviii.

[4]Sheldrake, *Presence of the Past*, p. xix.

[5]Sheldrake, *Presence of the Past*, p. 132.

[6]Julian Jaynes, *The Origins of Consciousness and the Breakdown of the Bicameral Mind* (Boston: Houghton Mifflin, 1976), p. 84

[7]Jaynes, *Origins of Consciousness*, p. 79.

[8]C. G. Jung, *Psychology and Religion: West and East* (New York: Pantheon, 1958), p. 456.

[9]Jung, *Psychology and Religion*, p. 259.

[10]Jung, *Psychology and Religion*, p. 556.

[11]William James, *The Varieties of Religious Experience: A Study of Human Nature* (New York: Random House, 1902), p. 498.

[12]C. G. Jung, *The Archetypes and the Collective Unconscious* (New York: Pantheon, 1959), p. 164.

[13]C. G. Jung, "The Psychology of the Unconscious," in *Two Essays on Analytical Psychology* (New York: Pantheon, 1953), p. 108.

[14]Erich Neumann, *The Origins and History of Consciousness* (Princeton: Princeton University Press, 1970), p. 414.

[15]Richard Leakey, *Origins Reconsidered: In Search of What Makes Us Human* (New York: Little, Brown, 1992), p. 92.

[16]Antonio R. Damasio, *Descartes's Error: Emotion, Reason and the Human Brain* (New York: Putnam's, 1994), p. 252.

[17]Paul D. MacLean, *The Triune Brain in Evolution: Role in Palocerebral Functions* (New York: Plenum Press, 1990), p. 578.

[18]Robert Lee Hotz, "Study: Brain's 'God Module' May Affect Religious Intensity," *Los Angeles Times*, October 29, 1997, p. 6.

[19]V. S. Ramachandran, *Phantoms in the Brain* (New York: William Morrow, 1998), p. 183.

Chapter 3: Neurostatic Representations

Conversion to the Secret Wisdom of the Culture

Socialization is normal and necessary for growing up. It is acquired by learning and unlearning, which includes being conditioned or converted to the culture's secret wisdom or religion. The word *religion* comes from the ancient Latin *religo*, which meant "to bind." The idea is that we bond our lives in common obligation with others, in the process giving power to the religious organization.

Where did the group or larger religious organization get its means of common obligation or secret wisdom, whereby it is able to condition or convert its individual members for its own exclusive purposes by collective bonding? The power comes from individuals who are on a path of their own, seeking and finding for themselves. After they have had an experience of their own wholeness, they attract followers who want to know the meaning of life. The followers identify within themselves what they see as their spiritual role model. Eventually, the group may expand into a cult, and later an accepted religion. What Jung said about the Mass being a process to bring wholeness or completeness to individuals, or what he called the individuation process, could be said about religion in general:

> The Mass is the summation and quintessence of a development which began many thousands of years ago and, with the progressive and deepening of consciousness, gradually made the isolated experience of specifically gifted individuals the common property of a larger group. The underlying psychic process remained, of course, hidden from view and was dramatized in the form of suitable "mysteries" and "sacraments," these being reinforced by religious teachings, exercises, meditations, and acts of sacrifice.[1]

What religions do is give their members connection or identity with a group in exchange for a limited amount of Neurostatic experience via conversion. They indirectly complete the wholeness of each member and provide an exclusive belief system, which is supported by rhythm and music, incense and wine, rituals and ceremonies, buildings and spaces, and other all-encompassing metaphors and symbols. To outsiders, the metaphors and symbols probably mean little and are harmless. However, the converted, who have accepted the group's representations for needs within themselves may be ready to set down their lives for these metaphors and symbols. If we learn from an early age to be part of a group—or, conversely, if we are deprived of religious associations in our formative years—we may easily, and perhaps unavoidably, give our brain functions over to an organization. Perhaps the future will provide some practical way of assisting people through the process of self unity without surrendering their identities to the purposes of organizations.

Several writers, including Arthur Koestler, have suggested that a drug or pill should be developed to satisfy the human need for spirituality or completeness without all the madness and manipulation that attend group religion.[2] Most people think of spiritual striving as involving participation in something beyond themselves. The reality, however, is that spirituality is already within us, and we don't need religious pills or organizations to deliver it to us from outside. Perhaps with our greater openness today to individual development, Neurostasis should be easier to find for those who persevere.

Individuals who have had the Neurostatic experience, or who comprehend what it involves without having experienced it, know something about the Neurostatic functions of the brain and to some extent understand the related metaphors and symbols in all their forms. If the Neurostatic experience comes from an outside source rather than from within, the experience is still real, but it is secondhand. It may be some time before we learn from neuroscience which brain functions and processes cause the seemingly mysterious experience that some people call religion and I call Neurostasis. In the meantime, we will have to rely on other sciences, including an anthropological understanding of the Neurostatic experience.

More than 2,500 gods and goddesses have been identified that people have believed in somewhere and sometime on this planet.[3] Undoubtedly, there are thousands more that are lost or unknown. These deities are like old wine in new bottles. The human need for them is an attempt, unknowingly and indirectly, to bring ourselves to ourselves through a cultural program.

As we try to understand this universe we live in, and as we begin to explore the nearby planets, it may seem strange that we have learned so much about the outer world and so little about the inner one. It is our inner world that makes us human.

The projection of our inner world out into our culture in the form of gods and goddesses has not greatly changed in the last ten to twenty thousand years except for the names of the characters. The stories are basically variations on a theme, but what we need to know more about is the underlying theme—unity, completeness, or Neurostasis. As Jung said, "self-realization…amounts to God's incarnation."[4]

Illustrations of Neurostasis-Derived Representations

The following pages present two types of illustrations: (1) expressions of individual development toward

Neurostasis; and (2) expressions of collective development utilizing Neurostasis. Both types give an impression of something happening that is not within our conscious control but embodies specific processes of our brain development. The illustrations are a small random group that I have selected in an attempt to provide a cross-section of cultural representations derived from the Neurostatic process, no matter how far they may be removed from the experiences of their original images. The illustrations include direct expressions of individuals and groups. The latter include mandalas, prayer rugs, a medicine wheel, a labyrinth, a swastika, and religious structures of various kinds. What is important about these illustrations is not how beautiful or interesting they are, but rather how they are a common reflection of the same Neurostatic source: brain unity activity.

The first two illustrations (Figures 5 and 6) are paintings from dreams that were important to Carl Jung. Years ago, when I was looking for a better understanding of my own experience, described in Chapter 1, I found that, under other names, Jung seemed to have had his own Neurostatic experience. He later came to work with many patients who also appeared to have had Neurostatic or religious experiences, for he stated:

> Among all my patients in the second half of life—that is to say, over thirty-five—there has

> not been one whose problem in the last resort
> was not that of finding a religious outlook.[5]

It is likely that many of Jung's theories will be further substantiated and may provide some basis for expansion of new discoveries when Neurostasis and its manifestations, such as sacred metaphors and symbols, are better understood physiologically. Jung himself speculated that within the subcortical part of the brain there is some physical basis for what I call Neurostatic images and he called mandalas, from the Sanskrit word for *circle*. "In the sphere of religious practices and psychology," he wrote, the mandala "denotes circular images, which are drawn, painted, modeled, or danced."[6] In a later reference, he added: "It [the mandala] is the 'uniting symbol' which epitomizes the total union of opposites. As such and in accordance with its paradoxical nature, it can only be expressed by means of symbols."[7]

Figure 5 reproduces a mandala painted by Jung in 1920, based on an image he had seen in a dream in 1914. This is an early example of a mandala painting done by Jung at a time when he was immersed in a "self-experiment" retreat that lasted for several years. It was a period for him of intense introversion, accompanied by self-discipline that included a form of meditation followed by strong emotion. Jung has written that "the years when I was pursuing my inner images were the most important in my life."[8] He later interpreted the mandala as a symbol of human wholeness or as the representation of a psychic centering process.

Jung's dreams ultimately led to development of the theory of individuation of the self, which was the centerpiece of his life's work, "the process by which individual beings are formed and are differentiated…, having for its goal the development of the individual personality. It is closely connected to the transcendent function."[9]

Figure 6 reproduces one of Jung's last mandala paintings, created in 1927, when he was fifty-two. It is based on an image that he had seen in a recent dream. This dream experience later confirmed the importance of the individuation process for Jung, giving him a sense that the goal of this process had been revealed. His years of self-experimental withdrawal were over. "One could not go beyond the center," he wrote. "Through this dream I understood that the self is the principle and the archetype of orientation and meaning."[10]

Jung's dreams were in some way derived from the same source as what I call Neurostatic experiences. All these types of images represent a basic force that can be found everywhere—in the cosmos, in the elements of matter, in the plant and animal worlds, and in objects and expressions created by our own self-consciousness. The first human representations of Neurostatic images go back to Paleolithic times, long before the invention of the wheel. They are circular designs scratched onto rocks perhaps as

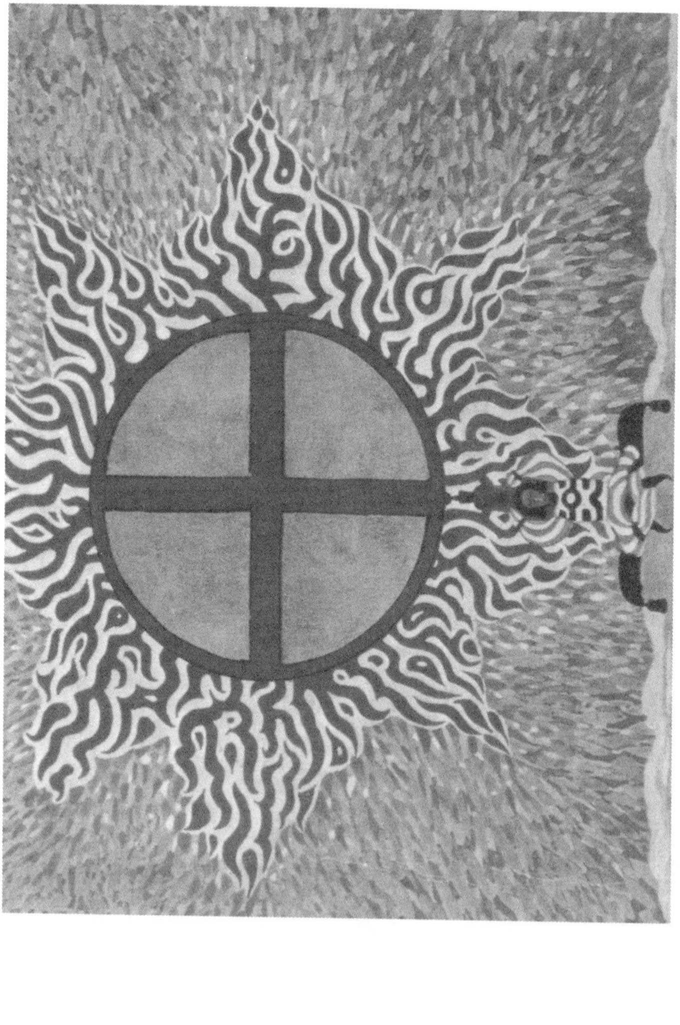

Figure 5:
Painting by Carl Jung: Untitled Mandala (1920)

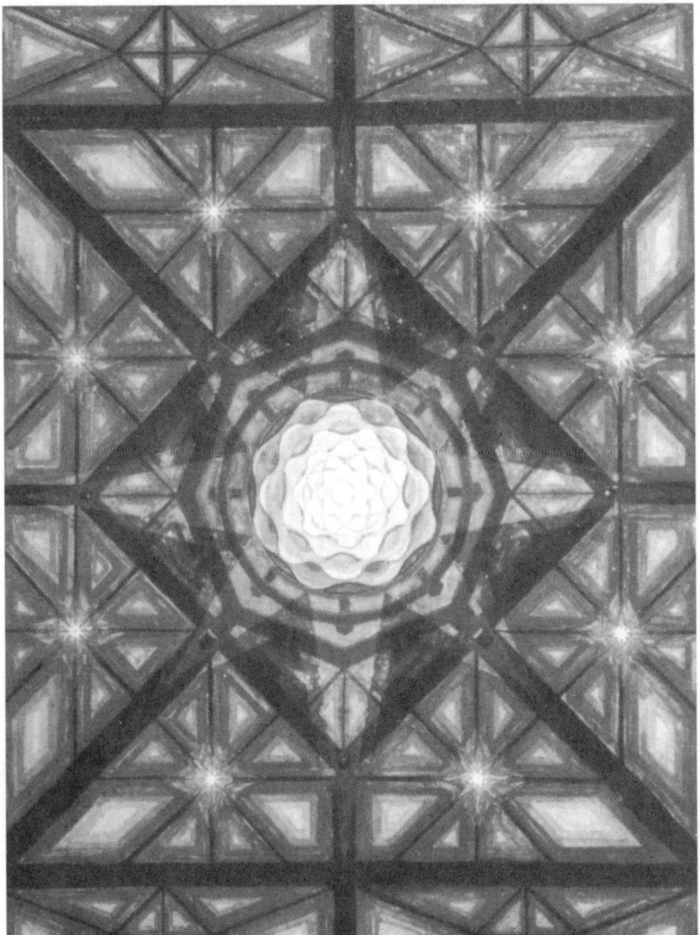

Figure 6:
Mandala: "Eternal Window" (1927)
Painting by Carl Jung

early as 30,000 years ago, possibly representing the sun, but more likely themselves. Unity images are found in all forms of spiritual groups and religions and are the underlying form of sacred structures.

Figure 7 reproduces "Mandala Universe" by Darryl Reanney, a molecular biologist at the Universities of New Zealand and Australia.[11] Reanney makes the following statements about his mandala:

> A highly speculative representation of the evolution of consciousness in a self-consistent, cyclic universe. At the beginning of the cosmos (the big bang), matter is in its simplest physical state, and intelligence does not exist. As space-time expands, matter begins an adventurous evolution that will lead to development of life systems. Out of that evolution grows the ability of the part to mirror the totality of the whole (consciousness).
>
> At this moment in evolution, consciousness is fragmented and rudimentary, handicapped by ignorance and confused by ego. All modes of consciousness, however, continue to exist in this "eternal" space-time structure, since the lowest and the highest levels are continuous with each other….
>
> In the mandala, the chain of cause and effect is continuous….
>
> The mandala shows how consciousness can be universal while at the same time frac-

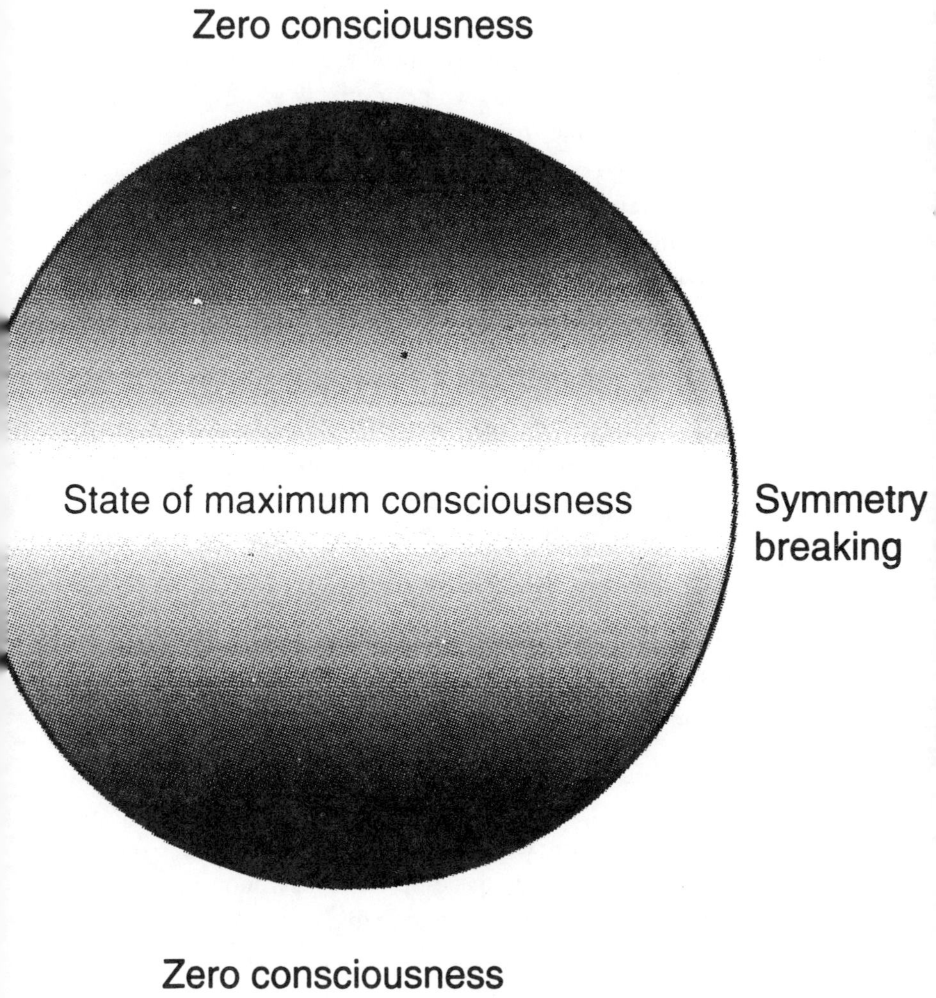

Figure 7:
"Mandala Universe" (1991)
by Darryl Reanney

tured into different reflecting crystals by ego boundaries....

In this mandala, there is no need for God to create (cause) the cosmos, since the act of creation is itself a result of its own prior effects....

Perhaps the mandala metaphor allows us to see why ego-death can free our consciousness from time, even at our present far from perfect stage of evolution.... All we can do is strive for the small ego-death that leads to that rare moment of insight so treasured by those who have experienced them....

This mandala sings to that consciousness that will continue to evolve into a truly supreme state in which it will be fully timeless and creatively free of all limitation."[12]

In attempting to deal with human consciousness and the quest for meaning, Reanney has provided an unusual expression of his Neurostatic inspiration:

I sketch out a mandala, a mythic symbol in the form of a Hawking space-time globe, a loop in time. Each pole is dark, symbolizing undifferentiated simplicity in a physical sense and total ignorance in a psychological sense. From the darkness, gradually, through evolution light is born and increases in strength. That light is information, the data stored in DNA code, and, in us, expressed as

> consciousness. The light of consciousness continues to brighten, reaching a maximum for reasons of pure symmetry at the equator of the space-time globe, after which it fades away again to reach another pole of darkness.[13]

Figure 8 reproduces "Impression of the Artist as Incorporeal Witness to the Center of the Universe" (1979), a sculpture by Robert Arneson.[14] The title appears to me to be a wonderful description of a Neurostatic experience. In connecting with the center of the universe, Arneson was connecting with the center of himself, or God.

Figure 9 shows an Islamic prayer rug with other "Persian" rugs in the background. These types of rugs, found throughout the Middle East and the Mediterranean area, are filled with Neurostatic representations, or what are commonly called medallions. They are known to have existed from the fifth century BCE. Prayer rugs, which are designed to face toward Mecca, are an integral part of the Islamic religion, which began with the quest of Mohammed (570–632 CE) to find the truth of God in the midst of many conflicting claims. In his late thirties, in a cave on Mt. Hira, Near Mecca, Arabia, Mohammed had a personal experience of God, or Allah. His revelations from that experience became the basis of the Koran. In the development of the Islamic religion, the representations of God were severely restricted to sacred geometry. This was particularly true in the design of mosques, which are very much Neurostatic representations.

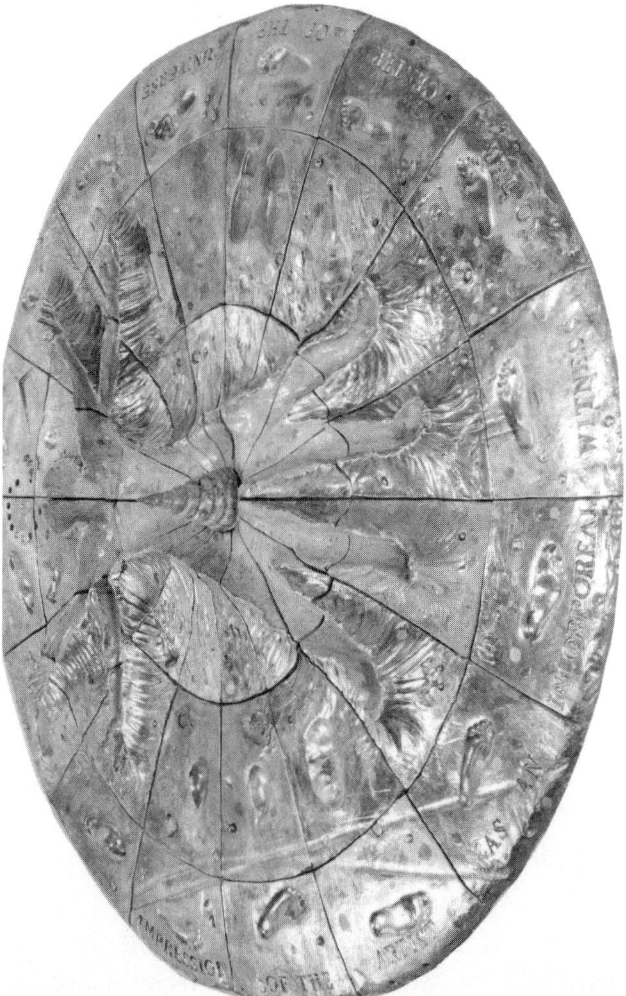

Figure 8:
"Impression of the Artist as Incorporeal Witness to the Center of the Universe" (1979)
by Robert Arneson
(Circular ceramic, 9½' diameter)

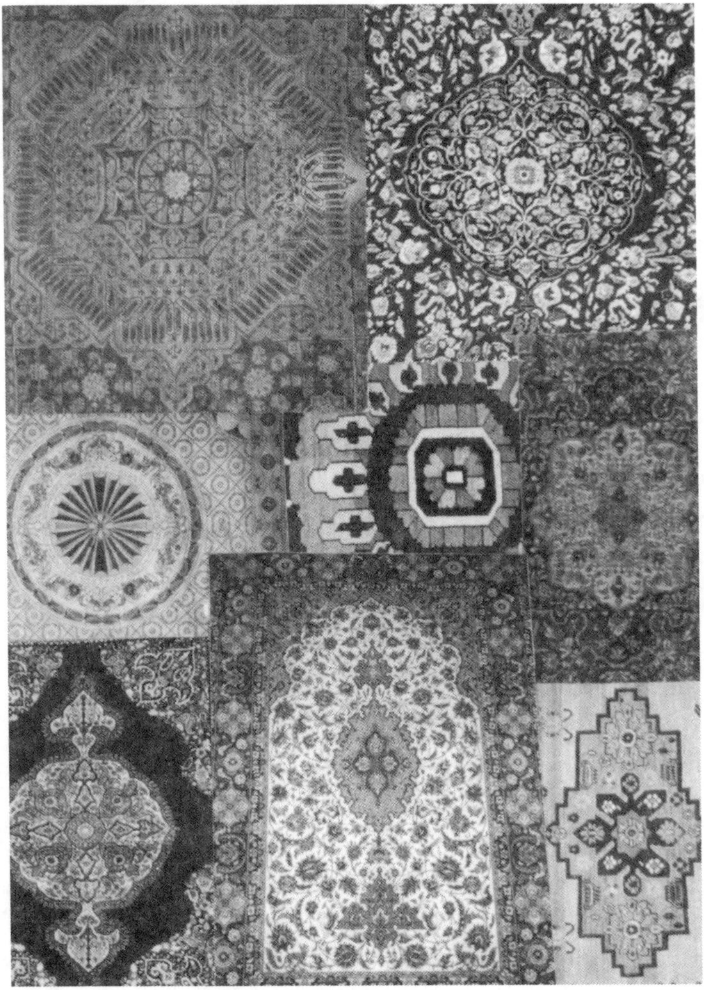

Figure 9:
Silk and Wool Persian Prayer Rug
Esfahan, Iran, 1986
4'-8" wide x 7' long

Figure 10 reproduces a mandala at the Temple Court in West Bhutan, representing the primary movement of the universe. Its circular form and concentric structure reflect the shape of the universe outside and the sense of perfection inside. As with all mandalas, concentrating on the form and content of this image aids in prayer and meditation, leading eventually to a complete sense of oneness within. Historically, the mandala symbol has been one of the most potent reflections of the human brain. Laughlin, McManus, and d'Aquili say of mandalas: "The coming together of neural structures at the transcendental warp seems to be a permanent stage in the perceiver's neurocognitive system. Its effects as a development transformation eventually permeate all cognition and experience."[15]

Figure 11 reproduces the Sri Yantra, one of the most common Hindu mystical symbols, most of which are related to the basic mandala design. The Sri Yantra is said to provide a means to find cosmic consciousness through meditation and prayer. The center is the starting point for finding this inner space.

Figure 12 is a Hindu mandala called "Bindu." It symbolizes the point of origin and return, drawing one toward its center. It has neither beginning nor end, nor is it positive or negative. It is unity.

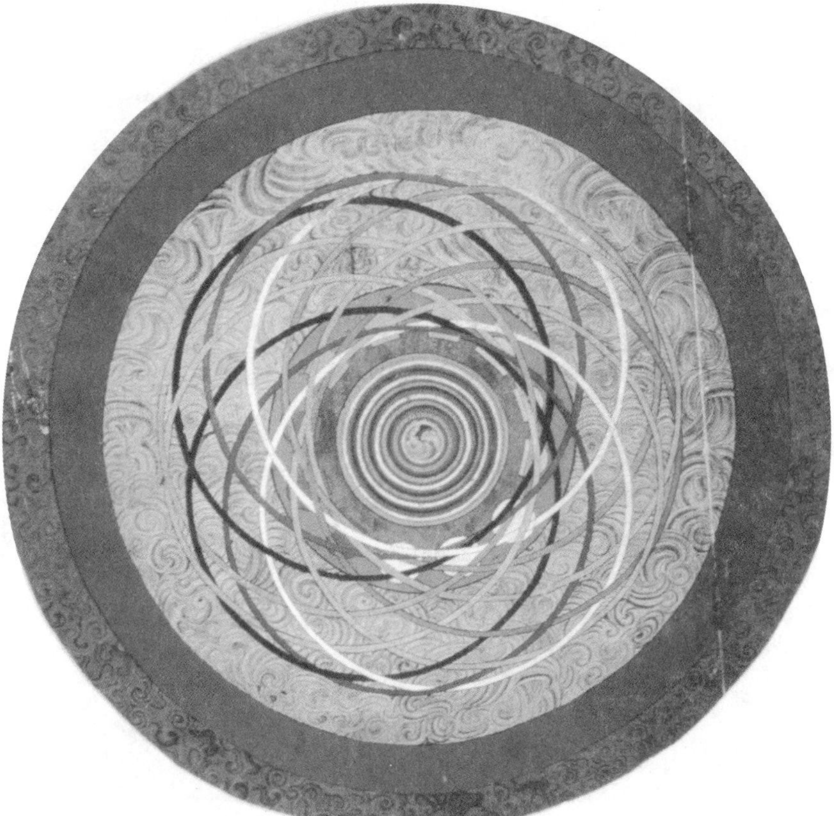

Figure 10:
Mandala from West Bhutan

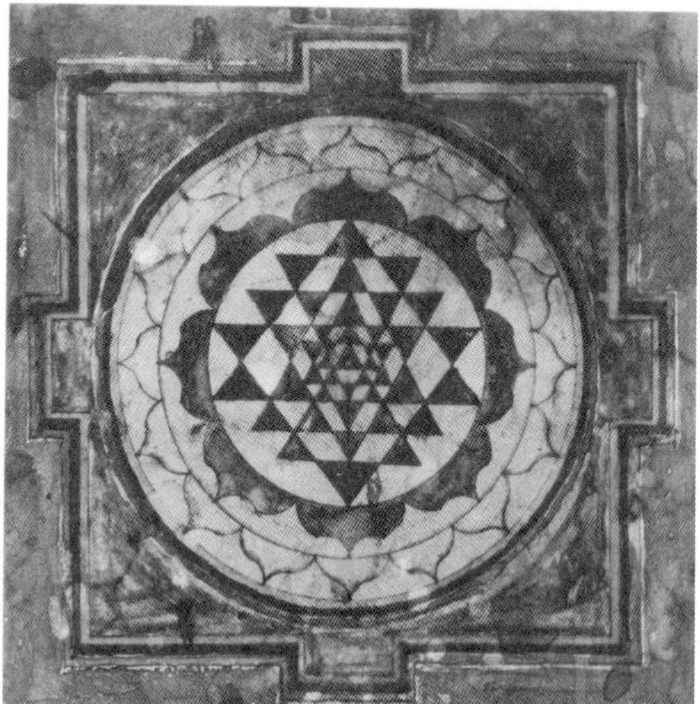

Figure 11:
The Sri Yantra, a Hindu Mandala from India

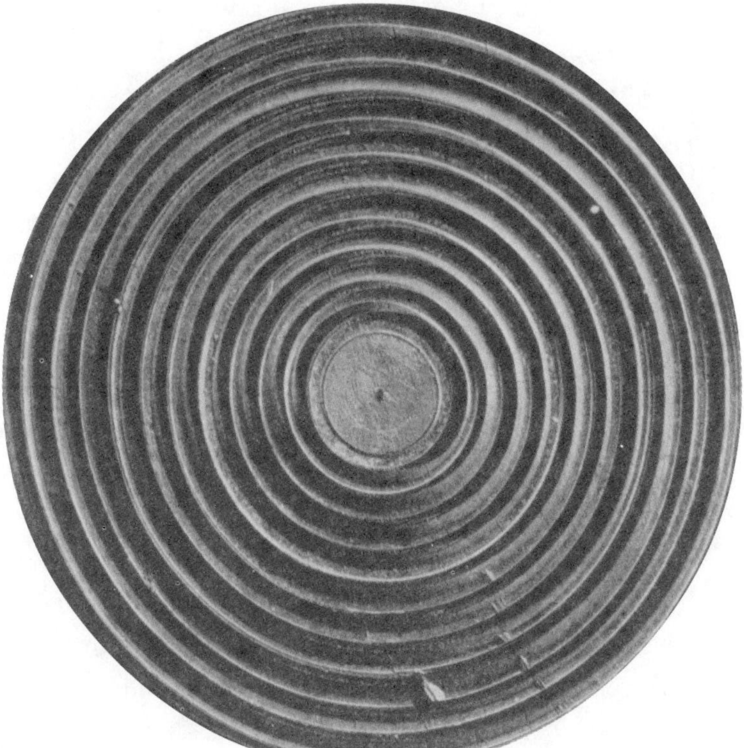

Figure 12:
Hindu Mandala Bindu

Figure 13 is a photograph of the remnant of an American Indian medicine wheel in the Bighorn Mountains of Wyoming. This Neurostatic image in stone, with a diameter of more than seventy feet, lies at an elevation of almost 10,000 feet. Its exact age is not yet known, but a similar monument due north in Canada has been determined to be approximately 5,000 years old.

American Indians comprehend time and life as circular rather than linear. Individuals are the center of their own circle, limitless and never-ending. Circles overlap and affect each other, interconnecting all humans and all other creatures. The circular concept is expressed in medicine wheels, which American Indians have used for thousands of years. Among other things, a medicine wheel is a tool to discover and maintain one's spiritual path. To be out of the circle of life is to be out of balance with one's self.

Medicine wheels are made in a variety of ways and sizes. Typically, a center is staked in the ground, and then a rope attached to the stake is used to draw a circle around it. The four directional points are then staked out on the circle. The wheel provides a focal point for centering the self by various ceremonies. The power of the circle is not in the telling but in the doing. It is not enough to simply look at the circle; one must experience it.

The medicine wheel is a symbol of God. It has a center or source that is motionless, while having direction and movement to and from that source. Today, each di-

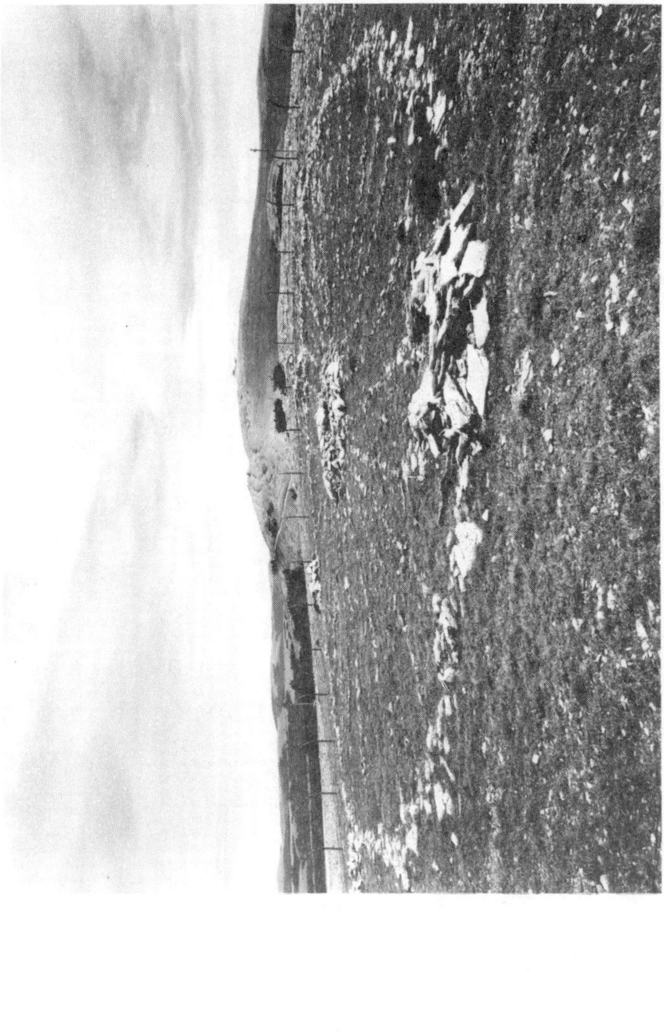

Figure 13:
Bighorn Medicine Wheel (Photo by Mark Junge)

rection has its color, animal, plant, mineral, and spirit keeper. There are also directions for such things as medicines, seasons, elements, and powers.

Light and the creative powers of the medicine wheel can radiate outward from or inward toward the center, source, or eye of God.

Figure 14 shows a monstrance, a piece of equipment once used prominently in Catholic rituals to display the "Host," the wafer used to symbolize the body of Jesus that was sacrificed—from the Latin *hostia*, "victim" or "sacrifice." The circular and radiant design from a center is one of many Neurostatic representations used by the Catholic Church. Some monstrances are so large that they can only be moved on wheels, such as in processions.

Figure 15 shows a Neurostatic representation in the form of a labyrinth, a piece of "sacred geometry." The California Pacific Medical Center, in San Francisco, California, where this picture was taken, apparently believes that a path to and from a central point may have value for spiritual and healing effects. It has recently become the first hospital in the United States to install a labyrinth on its grounds as part of its healing mission. The 36-foot wide circular walkway, one-third of a mile in length, is an exact replica of a labyrinth created eight hundred years ago by Benedictine monks on the floor of Chartres Cathedral in France. According to the hospital, the labyrinth is "a pattern that represents life..., a symbolic journey in the form of walking meditation."

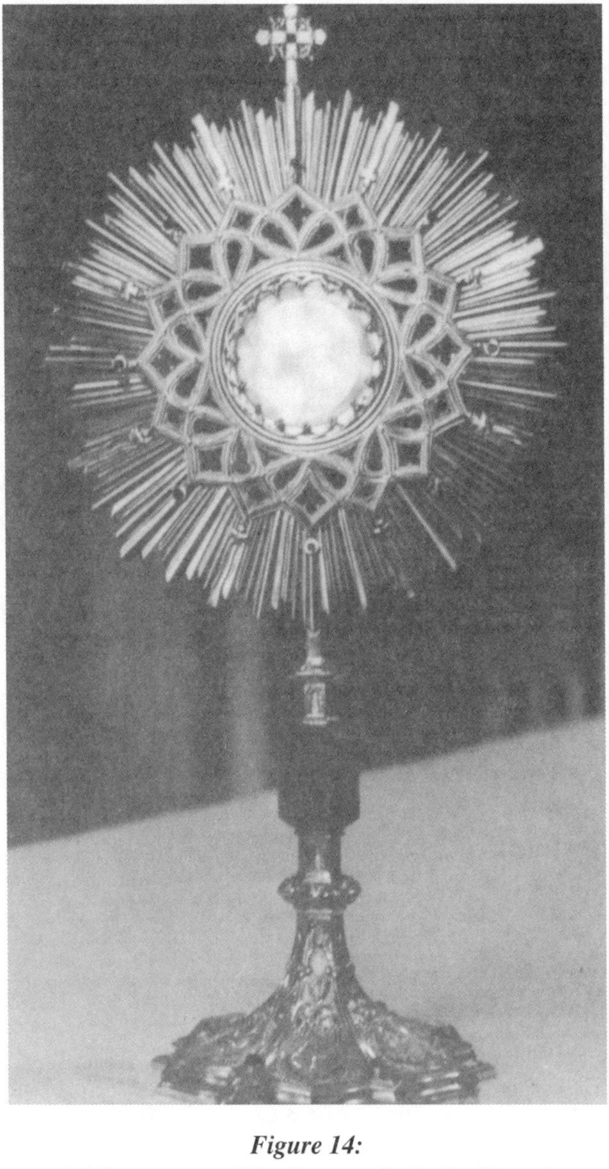

Figure 14:
A Monstrance of the Roman Catholic Church

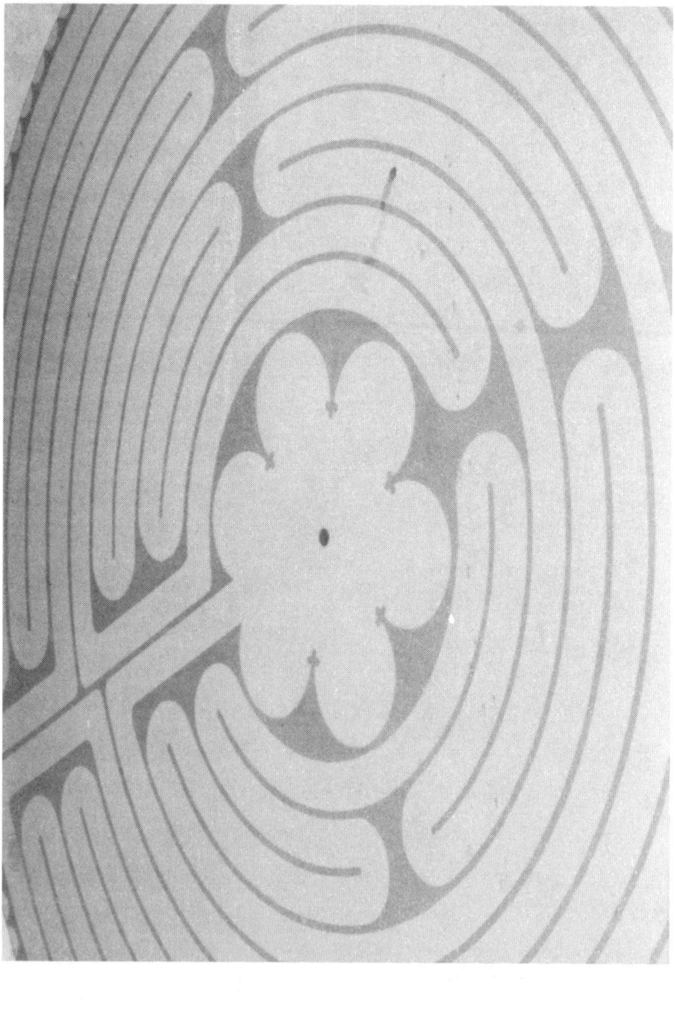

Figure 15:
Labyrinth at the California Pacific Medical Center
(Paint on concrete, 36' diameter)

Figure 16 shows the swastika, which was officially adopted as the emblem of Nazi Germany in 1935, when this photograph was taken. Between the first and second world wars, there were groups in Germany involved in the occult. The Nazi regime came to power from an occult group, with the supposed goal of achieving human perfection (including racial purification) by destroying the old decadent order. The Nazis were inspired by Nordic legends and the origins of the ancient Aryan people they considered their ancestors. The Nazi elite propagandized the German people into worshipping these reconstituted legends and myths. To that end, they borrowed the Hammer or Smasher symbol of the Norse God Thor, which was a swastika that he hurled, among other reasons, to create thunder and destroy anyone who offended him.[16]

At the end of the Second World War, because of the horror that the swastika had come to represent, its use in Germany was outlawed. We should be aware of how a representation for our inside can be taken and used for destructive and terrible purposes. In fact, the swastika is actually an ancient Neurostatic representation that has appeared in numerous parts of the world. In India, it is associated with the god Siva. The Sanskrit word *swastika*, or *svastika*, means "well-being" or "balance," but the design also indicates a turning movement. The swastika was also used in ancient Egypt, Greece, Troy, and Rome, and later in the Christian catacombs. The symbol has been found among the Celts in old Britain, in Pre-

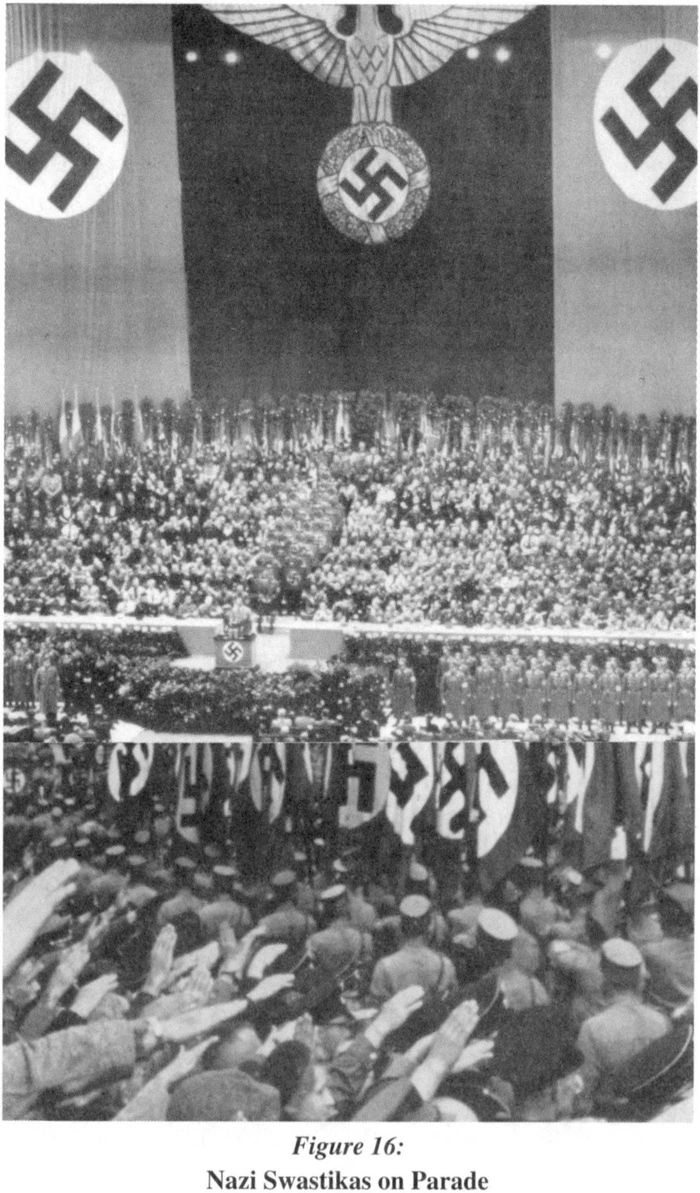

Figure 16:
Nazi Swastikas on Parade

Columbian America, on Easter Island, among American Indians, and in Japan, where it is known as Manji.

Figure 17 shows the literal and figurative center of Christianity in the Vatican interior, with the Pope standing above St. Peter's Tomb. The circular design is clearly a Neurostatic representation.

Stonehenge, pictured in Figure 18, one of the most recognizable monoliths from our prehistory, was constructed by the people of ancient England about 4,000 years ago. This massive oversized Neurostatic representation in stone was their attempt to make a connection within themselves, to make a connection with that which results from becoming self-conscious. It was a communal attempt to connect with a greater center source outside themselves.

The Stonehenge concentricity consisted of thirty large upright stones of about fifty tons each at the inner circle, bounded by a second circle of fifty-six similar stones, all capped by stone mantles. Other outlying circles had been mostly of other materials, such as timbers. There was earth mounding at the largest outside circle. In recent years, there have been attempts to show that Stonehenge was also constructed as an ancient calendar and as an astronomical observatory, to predict such events as eclipse cycles, seasonal phases, and sun and moon alignments. Throughout England today, some 3,000 stone circles have been identified. One of the largest, just found recently, had been made of very large timbers set up in nine concentric circles, with an outer diameter of nearly 500 feet.

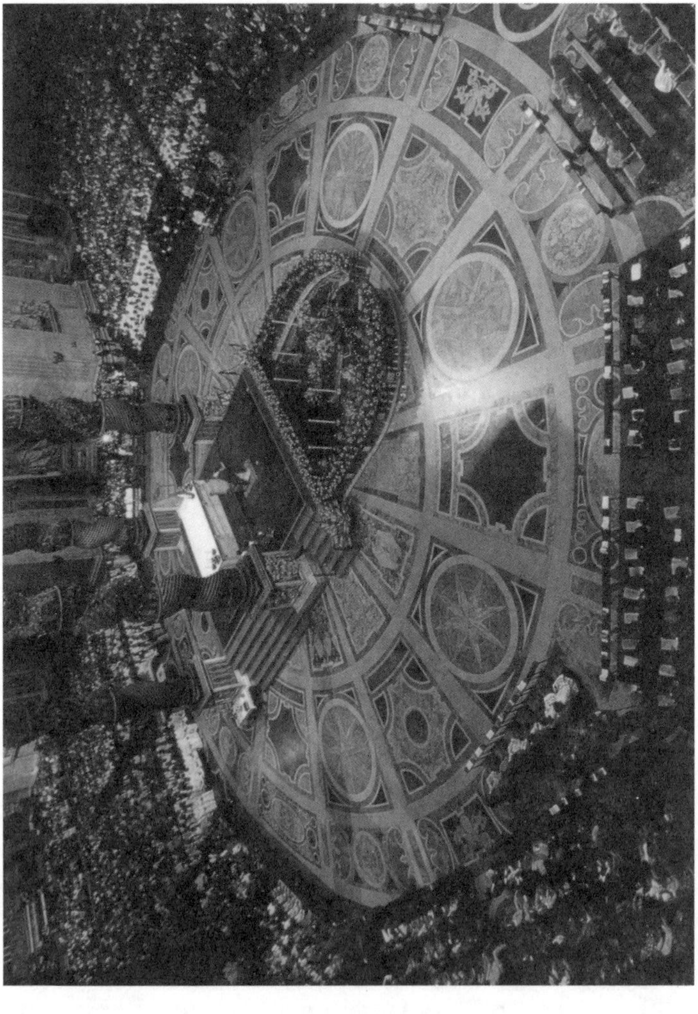

Figure 17:
St. Peter's Tomb in the Vatican

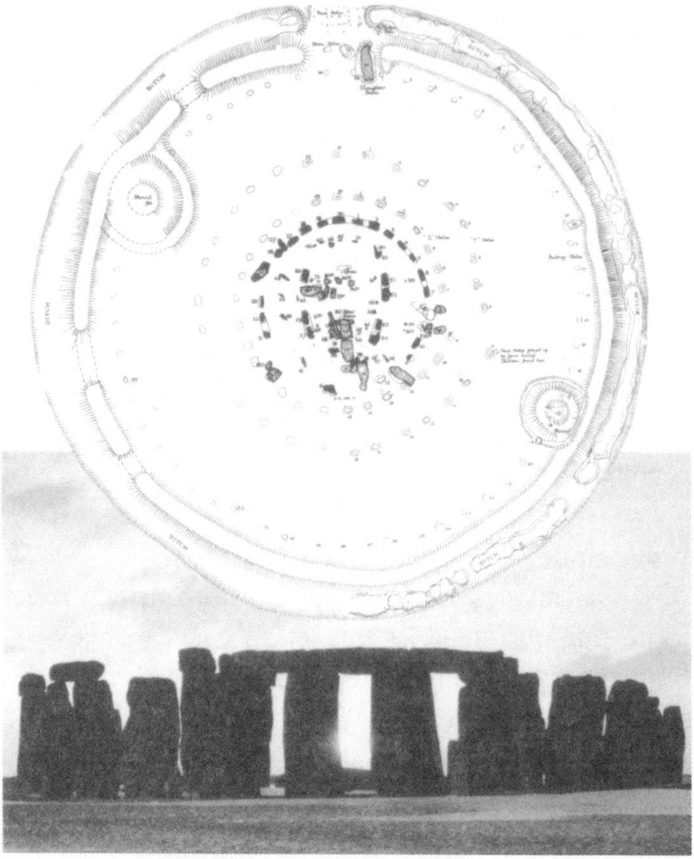

Figure 18:
Stonehenge

Buddhist shrines extend throughout the Far East. The one pictured in Figure 19, Boroabuour Stupa, is in Java. It rises like a terraced mountain in earth and stone. Nine levels of this Neurostatic representation lead up to a circular apex with a pinnacle center. Meditating worshippers move from the lower levels to the summit, progressing from the outer to the inner world.

Figure 20 gives a vision of Earth in space. It is a new experience for humanity to be able to see its home planet like a giant Neurostatic representation in the sky. For millennia we have placed ourselves in the center of the universe, and we have refused to budge, whether we belonged there or not. Now we will slowly learn deep within us that we and our Earth were never the center of the universe. This displacement from the center is assisted visually by the powerful image of Earth in space. Does anywhere in space provide the sacred and elusive center? Or is it everywhere, but mostly in our own brains?

Conclusion

The small scattering of examples shown on these pages expressing our unknown wholeness could be extended continuously in countless displays. Neurostatic representations are reflected in many and varied forms, from the vernacular to the intellectual, from the ideological to the commercial. What they represent is deep within us, interwoven through us, and colors our daily lives.

If our kind of consciousness has divided the world, and if it can only be made whole again when *we* are whole again, then that division is within us, within our brains.

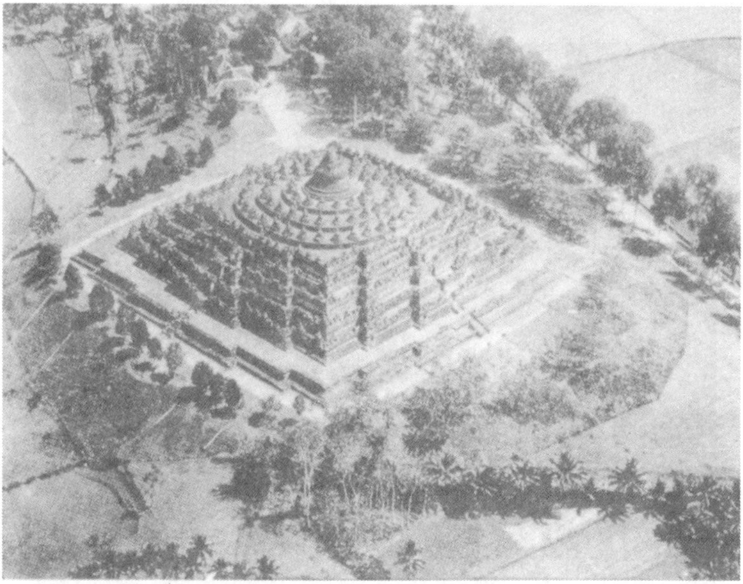

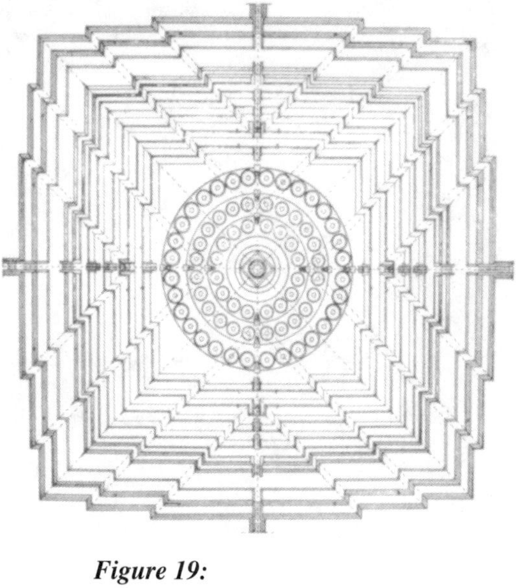

Figure 19:
Boroabuour Stupa in Java

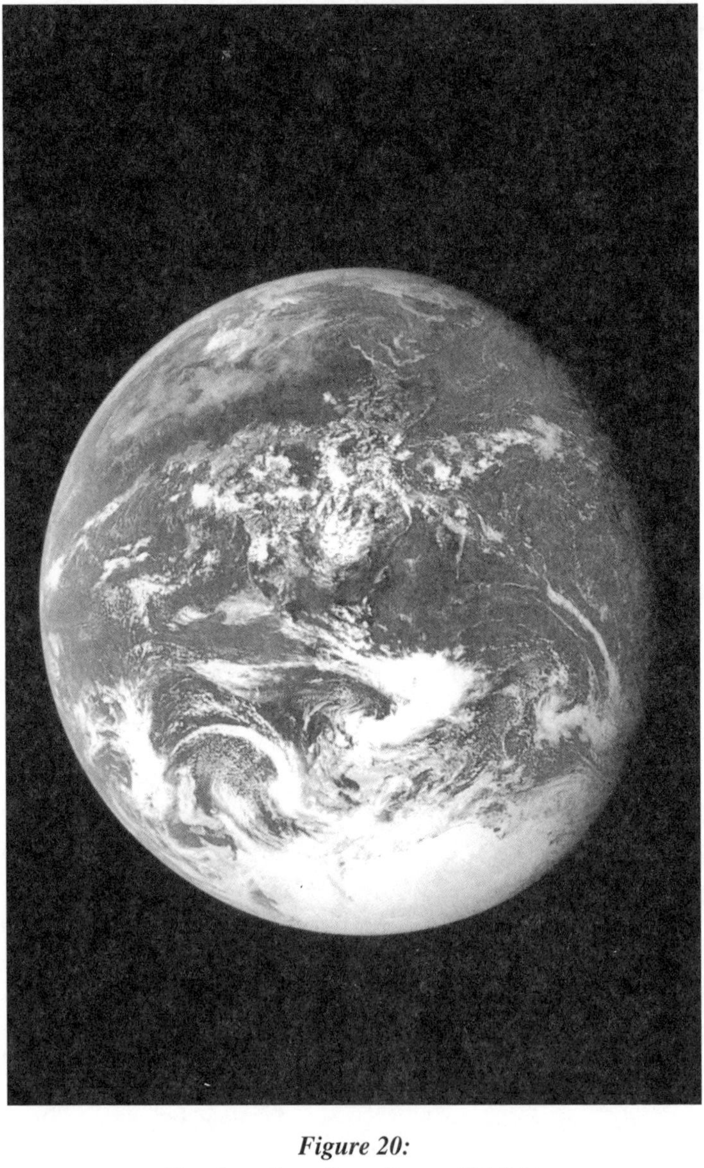

Figure 20:
Earth as Seen from Space (NASA)

Stephen Jay Gould, an extensive writer on evolutionary conditions and a paleontologist at Harvard University, has written that "we seem so driven to division by two, even in clearly inappropriate circumstances, that I must agree with several schools of thought in viewing our dichotomization more as an inherent mechanism of the brain's operation than any valid perception of external reality."[17] Until we know how and where within our brains we grow divided to be self-aware and later reunited to cause an experience of God, or what has been referred to here as Neurostasis, we need to appreciate and be more open to this experienceable and historical fact, in any form, for ourselves and others. We have to acknowledge that it is one of our main preoccupations.

There is no indication that within our brains the process referred to as Neurostasis is dissolving or fading away into our past. It is with us, and we need to look at this unique and natural gift that we have acquired or have been given, and consider what it means to us. The most critical factor in our everyday lives, and in human society in general, is what we have been calling transcendental or spiritual functions caused by the brain. But whatever they may be called, everything else follows these functions or conditions, to be resolved in some way, at least to some extent, sometime, somehow, and somewhere. Meanwhile, with this enigma, how do we live, how do we continue as individual human beings? In the early days of this country, it was claimed that each and every person, to the core, was given by the creator of everything, many gifts, including life, liberty, and the pursuit of happiness, while knowing of their opposites. From this claim, an agreement was instituted to provide for those intentions embodied in that document we call the United States Constitution. That same goal is still ours today—to determine if our agreements of the last two hundred years are still related to those original intentions for ourselves, for each and every one of us, and the world over, to become individual human beings.

Notes

[1]C. G. Jung, *Psychology and Religion: West and East* (New York: Pantheon, 1958), p. 295.

[2]See Arthur Koestler, *The Ghost in the Machine: The Urge to Self-Destruction—A Psychological and Evolutionary Study of Modern Man's Predicament* (New York: Macmillan, 1967), p. 337.

[3]Michael Jordan, *The Encyclopedia of Gods: Over Twenty-Five Hundred Deities of the World* (New York: Facts on File, 1993).

[4]Jung, *Psychology and Religion*, p. 157.

[5]Jung, *Psychology and Religion*, p. 334.

[6]C. G. Jung, *The Archetypes and the Collective Unconscious* (New York: Pantheon, 1959), p. 387.

[7]C. G. Jung, "Psychology of the Transference," in *The Practice of Psychotherapy: Essays on the Psychology of the Transference and Other Subjects* (New York: Pantheon, 1954), p. 264.

[8]C. G. Jung, *Word and Image* (Princeton: Princeton University Press, 1979), p. 66.

[9]C. G. Jung, *Psychological Types* (Princeton: Princeton University Press, 1971), pp. 448–449.

[10]Jung, *Word and Image*, p. 91.

[11]Darryl Reanney, *After Death: A New Future for Human Consciousness* (New York: William Morrow, 1991), p. 238.

[12]Reanney, *After Death*, pp. 238–241, 245.

[13]Reanney, *After Death*, p. 238.

[14]Robert Arneson, "Impression of the Artist as Incorporeal Witness to the Center of the Universe" (1979), 9½' diameter, ceramic. Estate of Robert Arneson/Licensed by VAGA, New York, NY.

[15]Charles D. Laughlin, Jr., John McManus, and Eugene G. d'Aquili, *Brain, Symbol, and Experience: Toward a Neurophenomenology of Human Consciousness* (New York: Columbia University Press, 1990), p. 333.

[16]Harold Bayley, *The Lost Language of Symbolism* (New York: Barnes & Noble, 1951), p. 121.

[17]Stephen Jay Gould, *Questioning the Millennium* (New York: Random House, 1997), p. 30.

Chapter 4:
Our Brains' Answer

How to Have a Religious (Neurostatic) Experience

Hopefully, the preceding three chapters have helped to explain why we have religious experiences and have described some of their power. These are experiences of brain images that come to consciousness to cause meaning for your life and to make you an ongoing completed human. You come to realize yourself as a whole, related to a whole. The experiences place you in a natural relationship with sex, money, power, life's games, and how to live your life.

The suggestions below are for those persons, most likely eighteen and older, who are sufficiently established as individuals to have a good sense of themselves and to be able to operate within the rules of the greater community. At some time, we have all had questions about life that were unanswerable. We have probably also had feelings that, since our encapsulated human world is limited to our awareness, that awareness may not be all that there is. In all likelihood, we have had occasional glimpses, flashes, or silences from within that have left behind a mystery.

The sure way to have a religious (Neurostatic) experience is not the easy way. The easy way is to get it secondhand from an organized group. The sure way is to get it from within yourself. As can be seen in the previous pages, we are only just beginning to realize that the brain functions in a way that causes religious (Neurostatic) experiences. However, we have yet to discover the factual information to confirm those functions, and so having a religious (Neurostatic) experience continues to be a difficult matter to deal with, as it always has been. Our religious (Neurostatic) experience for our wholeness cannot happen unless it is consciously self-caused or self-prodded or self-influenced. The way to yourself, the way to become whole, the way to God, is to trust yourself to give yourself to yourself. You must seek the answer of your greater self from your own experience. For this you cannot accept others' programs or experiences as your own.

There is no warranty for this process. There comes a time for each of us when our brains are physically ready for such an event. Self-consciousness, which is the main resistance to this experience, has to be ready and available to reactivate our original wholeness, so that our brains are renewed with unity images. It is unfortunate that even though we have had self-consciousness for quite a while, there has been no development of directions about how to deal with it, and no overall common understanding of that part of the brain or consciousness that gives us what we call religious experiences. The religious (Neurostatic) experience is important to make us completely human, since it allows the once-in-a-lifetime opportunity, as well as necessity, to be recentered within ourselves for our greater selves to receive the natural meaning of life.

Our history of religious experiences, including my own and those of my contemporaries, has given credence to these experiences. But if they are not approached in a spirit of openness to yourself, no amount of talking and no variety of methods will help you to have a religious (Neurostatic) experience. If you desire more how-to techniques, you should see additional sources, of which there are many. But realize that such books are almost always directed toward metaphorically and symbolically replacing your center with their message.

Ten Steps to Yourself

Here are some suggestions for how to have a religious (Neurostatic) experience. They are not instructions but the parameters of the ancient wisdom, "Seek and you will find," "Knock and it will open." You have to search and ask the questions that have been asked for thousands of years. Concentrate and make yourself receptive to yourself. There is no program other than yourself.

1. If possible, allow for a period of time—it could be six months, it could be a year, it could be two years—to find the answer, to find God within. We are all different in this regard, but it takes time for our brains to make adjustments to completion and for our self-consciousness

to allow for that completion. It is unlikely that you will be able to take passengers along, so be prepared to go it alone. This is appropriate because this will be a time for yourself. The traditional religious programs would take less time, and you would be part of a specific message of a specific community, but the experience would not be directly of and for yourself.

2. Dedicate this comparatively short time of your life to your life. Give your whole being to this endeavor, because nothing less will do. Be prepared to give up almost everything and travel light, because you are entering a world that previously you have only heard about or perhaps rarely peeked into. If you are going to dedicate yourself to this process, only *you* can do it. Getting advice will not do it, and a guide or helper cannot do it for you. The experience cannot be done for you. It is not necessary to believe anything except in yourself and life.

3. Find a place of minimal distraction and diversion. It should be comfortable and have easy access to reading materials and music. You need what works from your interior world, not your exterior world, such as television. This will be a time to withdraw from the outer world (to which you will return later), while continuing to maintain a balance between your inner and outer worlds. Begin to practice with your own thoughts of who and what you are, and trust yourself. Reflect on your problems or troubles so that you can feel their pressure, and then attempt to resolve them.

4. Concentrate and hold on to yourself. Be tough and patient with yourself. Drugs are not helpful overall and tend to be a sidetrack. Things such as sleep and nutrition deprivation and other kinds of self-torture are not necessary. To the extent possible, keep your senses fresh and open. It is self-awareness that you are working with.

5. Lay yourself open to yourself and trust completely in what you are doing. Test yourself by questioning *everything*, not just some things, and do not use other people's answers. Where did you come from, and where are you going? What are you, and why are you? Do you know how real your answers are? Can you feel their validity and tentatively trust the answers? Can you give answers to questions that have no answer? Go for the solution, even if it seems that there is no solution.

6. Even though you may become more contemplative, maintain contact with others. Support or discussion groups can be helpful. You may find it useful to be associated with a cultural group such as in a church, university, or museum. You might become acquainted with someone older, or with someone in a process similar to yours, or with someone with whom you simply can talk easily. Approach your life as an experiment.

7. Primarily, this is a time for searching, to see if life has meaning. Press yourself to find the meaning of your own existence. No one can give you the answer. Make an agreement with yourself not to accept anyone else's answer, because your brain is as capable as any to make these determinations.

8. Follow the search wherever it goes. In this special process, read or listen to whatever attracts you. Do not force yourself to comprehend something that is not interesting. At the same time, read, discuss, reflect, meditate, contemplate, dream, and experiment. Stretch yourself and go deeper. Relax and use self-discipline on the way to your core. Also use common sense.

9. This is a rare instance in your life to be completely natural with yourself, to be confident in what you are doing. If you have feelings that your survival may be in question, persevere, for your brain is working for life, for bringing together. Give yourself time.

10. It has been a while since you were born, when your brain began its development to be incomplete—this while causing and allowing your separate self-conscious individuality to grow and become mature. (The I-ness is not the whole self.) You can thank your unwholeness for permitting you to know that you exist. Once your I-ness is in place, your brain has a natural inclination, direction, and disposition to reestablish its original condition. Therefore, when you don't expect it, your brain will give you what is usually called a "religious experience." We do not yet have a pill or similar means to get there, so there are no real shortcuts to yourself. The only path to religious experience is to take the steps I have enumerated above. If, within the time you have set aside, you have not been able to reach the core of your being for a religious (Neurostatic) experience, then you should probably take

a break and give yourself over to a familiar traditional religious group. Perhaps, that group will be able to provide a substitute for your center, at least for a while, to assist you in returning from your withdrawal. If you got through stages 7 or 8, and struggled with 9 or 10, you have done something remarkable and are a better and more complete person for it. Beyond basic survival, this striving to complete ourselves is what human life is all about. It's in the doing.

Chapter 5: Summary and Hypothesis

The Purpose of Religious (Neurostatic) Experience

This book was written to bring to your attention that it is our brains that bring to our consciousness what we experience as religious (Neurostatic) experience. It seems that we are at the beginning level of human consciousness, which allows development of our own selves by ourselves. There is only one primary purpose of having a religious (Neurostatic) experience, and that is to complete our brain development. That completion includes several new realizations. Among them are:

1. The realization of unity fulfillment.

2. The realization of a natural and largely nonverbal understanding of life.

3. The realization of one's part in and empathy with everything.

We have a physiological readiness and necessity for religious (Neurostatic) experience. This readiness and necessity allow us to become complete as humans. Contrarily, we also have a self-consciousness that induces religious (Neurostatic) experience. What we perceive as our wholeness, or God, is a natural process that occurs in the brain. It overwhelms our everyday consciousness with unity images that give us a sense of completion. This experience then gives us an innate understanding of the meaning of life. Our fellow nonhuman creatures on Earth are not bothered with self-consciousness, since, as we did for a long time, they maintain their in-built consciousness system intact without it—and therefore without religion or Neurostasis. They are not complicated with incompleteness or self-consciousness to cause God or the experience of Neurostasis.

One implication of Neurostasis is that we begin to understand how the brain works for its completion—that is, we understand how God has been coming to us. When the physical basis of Neurostasis is factually known, life on Earth will slowly change for a new kind of human.

Underlying Ideas of the Neurostatic Experience

There are several ideas that underlie my basic concept of Neurostasis, ranging from assumptions to facts. I list them here to provide a brief overall summary of what I am proposing.

1. Although it is not well understood, there is an actual experience, which has aftereffects. It has a profound effect on our inner life. The human brain has a built-in

regulatory system related to consciousness. A process occurs within the brain that causes a more complete sense of self.

2. During this experience, one is overwhelmed by a conscious awareness of unifying forms or images of considerable light and energy. Although the experience is not under conscious control, it is a function of the brain that becomes conscious. In the past, it has sometimes been called a religious experience.

3. The experience only appears to occur once in a lifetime, but all of one's subsequent life is related to it. All living things strive to be what they are intended to be. Symbols and metaphors abound attempting to show this.

4. The experience has the same origins as *all* spiritual and transformational experience. It is a common and shared experience. It gives understanding and meaning to one's life. It also allows understanding of religious and other social organizations.

5. The necessity of this experience has resulted from the brain's longtime adaptation for a self-aware consciousness. As a result, there are brain processes that remain in effect undeveloped—or rather, during maturation these processes are held in some type of organic suspension.

6. During the first part of our lives, we evolve to grow unwhole until there is sufficient individual development to establish and maintain self-awareness and identity. Upon maturity this arrangement can incorporate the previous undevelopment within our brains to bring to con-

sciousness unifying visual images that have a profound emotional impact upon us.

7. The primary result of this experience is a sense of completion or unity. This is followed by change to the individual, with positive aftereffects that allow one to have an innate understanding of the meaning of life. It is sometimes identified as a religious or spiritual experience. It is often described as oneness with something outside ourselves, sometimes called God. Since we do not yet have actual factual data or a common language about our inner lives, this experience will likely continue to be misunderstood by most people. That will change when it is more generally acknowledged that it is our brains that bring this experience to consciousness.

The Hypothesis of Neurostasis or God Within

Neurostasis may be the basis of our humanity. It has a neurophysiological basis that is not yet fully understood, but occurs in at least three steps.

Step 1: At a certain point in the development of our adult self-consciousness, we begin to need compensation for the lack of our overall brain development. This need for compensation combines with various kinds of stress to cause Step 2.

Step 2: Stress can activate those subcortical elements or processes that are related to the whole brain. This activation may be related directly to the integrative and unifying functions of the brain. This dynamic activation or unification within our brains leads to unity images in our consciousness.

Step 3: The experience concludes with aftereffects that include a sense of oneness, wholeness, or God. One becomes, in effect, a complete human being with a new understanding of the meaning of life.

Conclusion

It will likely be some time before my hypothesis can be factually verified. Even so, people will continue to have Neurostatic experiences in many and varied forms, under varied names, collectively and individually. What I call Neurostasis may or may not be recognized in the immediate future by researchers in the brain sciences, but that will not change the ordinary human need to deal with our helplessness when we face ourselves.

The historical evidence of Neurostasis, or religious experience, extends back thousands of years, with countless participants and witnesses. To add to this knowledge in the contemporary world, one could establish a national registry to correlate all experiences of this type, thereby providing a statistical basis for its reality. One indirect attempt at this was made in the 1960s by Abraham Maslow, who encouraged individuals to provide him information about their so-called "peak experiences."

We may be in the beginnings of a glimmer of understanding of how the brain operates. Until recent years, there has been a tacit agreement among religious organizations, academicians, and researchers to keep religion or any knowledge about consciousness separate from science. It was thought that the "scientific method," being limited to determinism and material matters, could not be involved with spiritual matters. Science provides a higher level of consciousness than any other form of human endeavor, but it is missing a big part of the story—for example, the mysteries of memory and emotions, the nature of self and how we became human, and the meaning of life itself. It is time to know where our spiritual knowledge comes from so that we can survive on this planet. If we make scientific efforts to obtain such knowledge, that will help to raise us to a new level of common awareness. If our search for knowledge does not include the reality of all aspects of being human, including why we are spiritual, we could be heading toward a new kind of dark age.

This short book is intended to be read quickly. It is a way to convey what my experience means to me, what it may mean to you, and perhaps what it may ultimately mean to all of us. If you are a life seeker or want to be, this book should provide some idea about what you are seeking. Your purpose has always been the same—to experience a greater sense of yourself in addition to your I-ness. You will achieve your purpose naturally if you persevere and your self-consciousness is ready. That is to say, if you are ready, you will experience the Neurostasis that your brain will give you. In some form or other, Neurostasis has always been happening to people all over the world, and it will continue to do so. It involves becoming a complete person and becoming human. Knowing this will not inhibit this necessary experience. In fact, it should help.

Bibliography

Atkins, Peter. *Creation Revisited: The Origins of Space, Time and the Universe*. New York: W. H. Freeman, 1992.

Balfour, Mark. *Sign of the Serpent*. London: Prism Press, 1990.

Bayley, Harold. *The Lost Language of Symbolism*. New York: Barnes & Noble, 1951.

Damasio, Antonio R. *Descartes's Error: Emotion, Reason and the Human Brain*. New York: Putnam's, 1994.

Dewey, John. *Experience and Nature*. New York: Dover, 1958.

Gould, Stephen Jay. *Questioning the Millennium*. New York: Random House, 1997.

Hotz, Robert Lee. "Study: Brain's 'God Module' May Affect Religious Intensity." *Los Angeles Times*, October 29, 1997, p. 6.

James, William. *The Varieties of Religious Experience: A Study of Human Nature*. New York: Random House, 1902.

Jaynes, Julian. *The Origins of Consciousness and the Breakdown of the Bicameral Mind*. Boston: Houghton Mifflin, 1976.

Jordan, Michael. *The Encyclopedia of Gods: Over Twenty-Five Hundred Deities of the World*. New York: Facts on File, 1993.

Jung, C. G. *The Archetypes and the Collective Unconscious*. New York: Pantheon, 1959.

Jung, C. G. *Mysterium Coniunctionis: An Inquiry into the Separation and Synthesis of Psychic Opposites in Alchemy*. New York: Pantheon, 1963.

Jung, C. G. *Psychological Types*. Princeton: Princeton University Press, 1971.

Jung, C. G. *Psychology and Religion: West and East*. New York: Pantheon, 1958.

Jung, C. G. "Psychology of the Transference," in *The Practice of Psychotherapy: Essays on the Psychology of the Transference and Other Subjects*. New York: Pantheon, 1954.

Jung, C. G. "The Psychology of the Unconscious," in *Two Essays on Analytical Psychology*. New York: Pantheon, 1953.

Jung, C. G. *Word and Image*. Princeton: Princeton University Press, 1979.

Koestler, Arthur. *The Ghost in the Machine: The Urge to Self-Destruction—A Psychological and Evolutionary Study of Modern Man's Predicament*. New York: Macmillan, 1967.

Laughlin, Jr., Charles D., John McManus, and Eugene G. d'Aquili. *Brain, Symbol, and Experience: Toward a Neurophenomenology of Human Consciousness*. New York: Columbia University Press, 1990.

Leakey, Richard. *Origins Reconsidered: In Search of What Makes Us Human*. New York: Little, Brown, 1992.

MacLean, Paul D. *The Triune Brain in Evolution: Role in Palocerebral Functions*. New York: Plenum Press, 1990.

Neumann, Erich. *The Origins and History of Consciousness*. Princeton: Princeton University Press, 1970.

Ramachandran, V. S. *Phantoms in the Brain*. New York: William Morrow, 1998.

Reanney, Darryl. *After Death: A New Future for Human Consciousness*. New York: William Morrow, 1991.

Sheldrake, Rupert. *The Presence of the Past: Morphic Resonance and the Habits of Nature*. Rochester, Vt.: Park Street Press, 1988.

Index

Adolescence, 10, 12, 15, 52
Adulthood, see Maturity
Amygdalae, 37
Aristotle, 51
Arneson, Robert, 83–84
Atkins, Peter, 45–46

Biology
as basis of Neurostasis, 67
as process, simple or complicated, 55
Bonding, human, 55, 71
Brain, ancient, 56
Brain-caused unity, 18, 56
Brainminding, 41
Brain's answer to life's meaning, xv, 107
Brainwashing, 38, 40

Cajal, Santiago Ramon y, 38
Carriers of life, 52
Center
and beyond, 77
and soul, 1, 9
as starting point, 86
elusiveness of, 100
enveloped in, 19
in children's art, 54
in Neurostatic images, 59
knowing, 15, 67
of Eden, 2, 3
of ourselves, 6
of singularity, xv
of the universe, 6, 83
or unifying effect, 18
source outside, 97
Cerebellum, 37
Children's art, 54
Community, 40, 55
Completeness
blind search for, 12
need for human, 38
realizations of, 8, 10, 118, 121
receptiveness to, 11
underlying theme of, 74
Completeness-consciousness, 33
Concentric patterns, 19
Consciousness, 1, 11, 18, 21, 23–24, 26, 32–33
Corpus callosum, 35
Cortex, 35
Culture, 6, 41, 48, 65, 71, 74

Damasio, Antonio, 66
Deep structure, 45–46
Descartes, René, 16
Dewey, John, 7
DNA, 39
Dreams, wide awake, 17
Drugs, 17, 3, 55, 73, 111

Eden, Garden of, xiii, 2–3, 65
Either/or thinking, 43
Evolution
and a new scientific concept, 46
and consciousness, 34, 41
and the Big Bang, xv
and the brain, 8, 44
metaphor of life as, 65–66

God (also see Neurostasis, Religion), 6, 8, 30-31, 50, 90, 103, 108–109, 116, 118

God in our brain
and Neurostasis, 6
experience of, 26, 41, 54, 66
Gould, Stephen Jay, 103
Groups, 6, 50, 53, 73, 117

Hindu symbols, 20
Hippocampi, 37
Homeostasis, 9, 43
Hypothalami, 37

Individuality, 52–54, 72–73, 103–104, 107, 117
Individuation, 72, 77
I-ness, 8, 10, 24–25, 32, 52–53, 65, 120

James, William, 56
Jaynes, Julian, 49
Jung, Carl, 20, 25, 53, 55, 58–59, 71–72, 75–79

Koestler, Arthur, 73

Labyrinths, 92, 94
Leakey, Richard, 64
Light, 17, 19, 25, 50–51, 58, 117
Limbic system, 66

MacLean, Paul, xiii, 66
Maslow, Abraham, 119
Maturity, 8, 11, 117
Metaphors
and experience, 25, 31
and Garden of Eden, 2
and inner life, 44–46
and psychobiological transformation, 5
and understanding, 1, 82
as cultural symbols, 39
harmlessness of, 72
meaning of, 48
Metaphors *(cont'd)*
universality of, 65
Morphic fields, morphic resonance, 46–47
Mumford, Lewis, 15

Nature, 23, 53
Neumann, Erick, 60
Neurochemicals, 8–9, 38
Neurophysiology
and completeness-consciousness, 33
and consciousness, 32
and Neurostasis, 118
and religious experience, 7
and self-consciousness, 33
and the brain, 68
Neurostasis (also see Religion)
and God, 8
and life, 10
and religious experience, 115–116
and wholeness, 8
experience of, 17–26, 30, 67
explanation of, 4, 7, 15, 17–26, 116–119
images of, 23, 25–26, 58–60, 74–75
need for, 32–33
Neurotransmitters, 38
Numbers, 46

Organizations, see Groups

Paleolithic Age, 77
Pavlov, Ivan, 38
Pituitary gland, 37
Primates, 64–65
Psychobiological transformation, 5

Radiance, see Light
Ramachandran, R. S., 67

Reanney, Darryl, 80–82
Religion (also see Neurostasis), 31, 71

Scientific method, 15, 120
Self, larger or greater, 7–8
Self-consciousness, 5, 10–11, 24, 29, 32–34
Self-healing, 20, 60
Self-identification, 8
Self-organization, 51
Self-resonance, 47–48
Sheldrake, Rupert, 46–47
Socrates, 55
Soul center, 1, 9
Sperry, Roger, 39
Stress, 8, 58, 118
Symmetry, bilateral, 61, 64
Synapse, 38

Thalami, 35
Transformations, 9, 58–59, 103, 117

Uniqueness, 2, 29
Unity, xv, 9–11, 17–18, 21, 54, 56, 118–119
Universal myths, 65
Unwholeness (also see Wholeness), 10–12, 112, 117

Wholeness (also see Unwholeness), 1, 10–12, 34, 50, 54–55, 71, 107–108, 116, 119